Mental Health Policy and Service Guidance Package

ORGANIZATION OF SERVICES FOR MENTAL HEALTH

World Health Organization, 2003

WHO Library Cataloguing-in-Publication Data

Organization of services for mental health.
(Mental health policy and service guidance package)

1. Mental health services - organization and administration
2. Community mental health services - organization and administration
3. Delivery of health care, Integrated
4. Health planning guidelines I. World Health Organization II. Series.

ISBN 92 4 154592 5
(NLM classification: WM 30)

Technical information concerning this publication can be obtained from:
Dr Michelle Funk
Mental Health Policy and Service Development Team
Department of Mental Health and Substance Dependence
Noncommunicable Diseases and Mental Health Cluster
World Health Organization
CH-1211, Geneva 27
Switzerland
Tel: +41 22 791 3855
Fax: +41 22 791 4160
E-mail: funkm@who.int

Printed in Singapore.

Acknowledgements

The Mental Health Policy and Service Guidance Package was produced under the direction of Dr Michelle Funk, Coordinator, Mental Health Policy and Service Development, and supervised by Dr Benedetto Saraceno, Director, Department of Mental Health and Substance Dependence, World Health Organization.

The World Health Organization gratefully thanks Dr Soumitra Pathare, Ruby Hall Clinic, Pune, India who prepared this module. Professor Alan Flisher, University of Cape Town, Observatory, Republic of South Africa, Dr Silvia Kaaya, Department of Psychiatry, Muhimbili Medical Centre, Dar es Salaam, Tanzania, Dr Gad Kilonzo, Department of Psychiatry, Muhimbili Medical Centre, Dar es Salaam, Tanzania, Dr Ian Lockhart, University of Cape Town, Observatory, Republic of South Africa and Dr Jesse K. Mbwambo, Department of Psychiatry, Muhimbili Medical Centre, Dar es Salaam, Tanzania also drafted documents that were used in its preparation.

Editorial and technical coordination group:

Dr Michelle Funk, World Health Organization, Headquarters (WHO/HQ), Ms Natalie Drew, (WHO/HQ), Dr JoAnne Epping-Jordan, (WHO/HQ), Professor Alan J. Flisher, University of Cape Town, Observatory, Republic of South Africa, Professor Melvyn Freeman, Department of Health, Pretoria, South Africa, Dr Howard Goldman, National Association of State Mental Health Program Directors Research Institute and University of Maryland School of Medicine, USA, Dr Itzhak Levav, Mental Health Services, Ministry of Health, Jerusalem, Israel and Dr Benedetto Saraceno, (WHO/HQ).

Dr Crick Lund, University of Cape Town, Observatory, Republic of South Africa, finalized the technical editing of this module.

Technical assistance:

Dr Jose Bertolote, World Health Organization, Headquarters (WHO/HQ), Dr Thomas Bornemann (WHO/HQ), Dr José Miguel Caldas de Almeida, WHO Regional Office for the Americas (AMRO), Dr Vijay Chandra, WHO Regional Office for South-East Asia (SEARO), Dr Custodia Mandlhate, WHO Regional Office for Africa (AFRO), Dr Claudio Miranda (AMRO), Dr Ahmed Mohit, WHO Regional Office for the Eastern Mediterranean, Dr Wolfgang Rutz, WHO Regional Office for Europe (EURO), Dr Erica Wheeler (WHO/HQ), Dr Derek Yach (WHO/HQ), and staff of the WHO Evidence and Information for Policy Cluster (WHO/HQ).

Administrative and secretarial support:

Ms Adeline Loo (WHO/HQ), Mrs Anne Yamada (WHO/HQ) and Mrs Razia Yaseen (WHO/HQ).

Layout and graphic design: 2S) graphicdesign
Editor: Walter Ryder

WHO also gratefully thanks the following people for their expert opinion and technical input to this module:

Dr Adel Hamid Afana	Director, Training and Education Department Gaza Community Mental Health Programme
Dr Bassam Al Ashhab	Ministry of Health, Palestinian Authority, West Bank
Mrs Ella Amir	Ami Québec, Canada
Dr Julio Arboleda-Florez	Department of Psychiatry, Queen's University, Kingston, Ontario, Canada
Ms Jeannine Auger	Ministry of Health and Social Services, Québec, Canada
Dr Florence Baingana	World Bank, Washington DC, USA
Mrs Louise Blanchette	University of Montreal Certificate Programme in Mental Health, Montreal, Canada
Dr Susan Blyth	University of Cape Town, Cape Town, South Africa
Ms Nancy Breitenbach	Inclusion International, Ferney-Voltaire, France
Dr Anh Thu Bui	Ministry of Health, Koror, Republic of Palau
Dr Sylvia Caras	People Who Organization, Santa Cruz, California, USA
Dr Claudina Cayetano	Ministry of Health, Belmopan, Belize
Dr Chueh Chang	Taipei, Taiwan
Professor Yan Fang Chen	Shandong Mental Health Centre, Jinan People's Republic of China
Dr Chantharavdy Choulamany	Mahosot General Hospital, Vientiane, Lao People's Democratic Republic
Dr Ellen Corin	Douglas Hospital Research Centre, Quebec, Canada
Dr Jim Crowe	President, World Fellowship for Schizophrenia and Allied Disorders, Dunedin, New Zealand
Dr Araba Sefa Dedeh	University of Ghana Medical School, Accra, Ghana
Dr Nimesh Desai	Professor of Psychiatry and Medical Superintendent, Institute of Human Behaviour and Allied Sciences, India
Dr M. Parameshvara Deva	Department of Psychiatry, Perak College of Medicine, Ipoh, Perak, Malaysia
Professor Saida Douki	President, Société Tunisienne de Psychiatrie, Tunis, Tunisia
Professor Ahmed Abou El-Azayem	Past President, World Federation for Mental Health, Cairo, Egypt
Dr Abra Fransch	WONCA, Harare, Zimbabwe
Dr Gregory Fricchione	Carter Center, Atlanta, USA
Dr Michael Friedman	Nathan S. Kline Institute for Psychiatric Research, Orangeburg, NY, USA
Mrs Diane Froggatt	Executive Director, World Fellowship for Schizophrenia and Allied Disorders, Toronto, Ontario, Canada
Mr Gary Furlong	Metro Local Community Health Centre, Montreal, Canada
Dr Vijay Ganju	National Association of State Mental Health Program Directors Research Institute, Alexandria, VA, USA
Mrs Reine Gobeil	Douglas Hospital, Quebec, Canada
Dr Nacanieli Goneyali	Ministry of Health, Suva, Fiji
Dr Gaston Harnois	Douglas Hospital Research Centre, WHO Collaborating Centre, Quebec, Canada
Mr Gary Haugland	Nathan S. Kline Institute for Psychiatric Research, Orangeburg, NY, USA
Dr Yanling He	Consultant, Ministry of Health, Beijing, People's Republic of China
Professor Helen Herrman	Department of Psychiatry, University of Melbourne, Australia

Mrs Karen Hetherington	WHO/PAHO Collaborating Centre, Canada
Professor Frederick Hickling	Section of Psychiatry, University of West Indies, Kingston, Jamaica
Dr Kim Hopper	Nathan S. Kline Institute for Psychiatric Research, Orangeburg, NY, USA
Dr Tae-Yeon Hwang	Director, Department of Psychiatric Rehabilitation and Community Psychiatry, Yongin City, Republic of Korea
Dr A. Janca	University of Western Australia, Perth, Australia
Dr Dale L. Johnson	World Fellowship for Schizophrenia and Allied Disorders, Taos, NM, USA
Dr Kristine Jones	Nathan S. Kline Institute for Psychiatric Research, Orangeburg, NY, USA
Dr David Musau Kiima	Director, Department of Mental Health, Ministry of Health, Nairobi, Kenya
Mr Todd Krieble	Ministry of Health, Wellington, New Zealand
Mr John P. Kummer	Equilibrium, Unteraegeri, Switzerland
Professor Lourdes Ladrido-Ignacio	Department of Psychiatry and Behavioural Medicine, College of Medicine and Philippine General Hospital, Manila, Philippines
Dr Pirkko Lahti	Secretary-General/Chief Executive Officer, World Federation for Mental Health, and Executive Director, Finnish Association for Mental Health, Helsinki, Finland
Mr Eero Lahtinen,	Ministry of Social Affairs and Health, Helsinki, Finland
Dr Eugene M. Laska	Nathan S. Kline Institute for Psychiatric Research, Orangeburg, NY, USA
Dr Eric Latimer	Douglas Hospital Research Centre, Quebec, Canada
Dr Ian Lockhart	University of Cape Town, Observatory, Republic of South Africa
Dr Marcelino López	Research and Evaluation, Andalusian Foundation for Social Integration of the Mentally Ill, Seville, Spain
Ms Annabel Lyman	Behavioural Health Division, Ministry of Health, Koror, Republic of Palau
Dr Ma Hong	Consultant, Ministry of Health, Beijing, People's Republic of China
Dr George Mahy	University of the West Indies, St Michael, Barbados
Dr Joseph Mbatia	Ministry of Health, Dar-es-Salaam, Tanzania
Dr Céline Mercier	Douglas Hospital Research Centre, Quebec, Canada
Dr Leen Meulenbergs	Belgian Inter-University Centre for Research and Action, Health and Psychobiological and Psychosocial Factors, Brussels, Belgium
Dr Harry I. Minas	Centre for International Mental Health and Transcultural Psychiatry, St. Vincent's Hospital, Fitzroy, Victoria, Australia
Dr Alberto Minoletti	Ministry of Health, Santiago de Chile, Chile
Dr P. Mogne	Ministry of Health, Mozambique
Dr Paul Morgan	SANE, South Melbourne, Victoria, Australia
Dr Driss Moussaoui	Université psychiatrique, Casablanca, Morocco
Dr Matt Muijen	The Sainsbury Centre for Mental Health, London, United Kingdom
Dr Carmine Munizza	Centro Studi e Ricerca in Psichiatria, Turin, Italy
Dr Shisram Narayan	St Giles Hospital, Suva, Fiji
Dr Sheila Ndyanabangi	Ministry of Health, Kampala, Uganda
Dr Grayson Norquist	National Institute of Mental Health, Bethesda, MD, USA
Dr Frank Njenga	Chairman of Kenya Psychiatrists' Association, Nairobi, Kenya

Dr Angela Ofori-Atta	Clinical Psychology Unit, University of Ghana Medical School, Korle-Bu, Ghana
Professor Mehdi Paes	Arrazi University Psychiatric Hospital, Sale, Morocco
Dr Rampersad Parasram	Ministry of Health, Port of Spain, Trinidad and Tobago
Dr Vikram Patel	Sangath Centre, Goa, India
Dr Dixianne Penney	Nathan S. Kline Institute for Psychiatric Research, Orangeburg, NY, USA
Dr Yogan Pillay	Equity Project, Pretoria, Republic of South Africa
Dr M. Pohanka	Ministry of Health, Czech Republic
Dr Laura L. Post	Mariana Psychiatric Services, Saipan, USA
Dr Prema Ramachandran	Planning Commission, New Delhi, India
Dr Helmut Remschmidt	Department of Child and Adolescent Psychiatry, Marburg, Germany
Professor Brian Robertson	Department of Psychiatry, University of Cape Town, Republic of South Africa
Dr Julieta Rodriguez Rojas	Integrar a la Adolescencia, Costa Rica
Dr Agnes E. Rupp	Chief, Mental Health Economics Research Program, NIMH/NIH, USA
Dr Ayesh M. Sammour	Ministry of Health, Palestinian Authority, Gaza
Dr Aive Sarjas	Department of Social Welfare, Tallinn, Estonia
Dr Radha Shankar	AASHA (Hope), Chennai, India
Dr Carole Siegel	Nathan S. Kline Institute for Psychiatric Research, Orangeburg, NY, USA
Professor Michele Tansella	Department of Medicine and Public Health, University of Verona, Italy
Ms Mrinali Thalgodapitiya	Executive Director, NEST, Hendala, Watala, Gampaha District, Sri Lanka
Dr Graham Thornicroft	Director, PRISM, The Maudsley Institute of Psychiatry, London, United Kingdom
Dr Giuseppe Tibaldi	Centro Studi e Ricerca in Psichiatria, Turin, Italy
Ms Clare Townsend	Department of Psychiatry, University of Queensland, Toowing Qld, Australia
Dr Gombodorjiin Tsetsegdary	Ministry of Health and Social Welfare, Mongolia
Dr Bogdana Tudorache	President, Romanian League for Mental Health, Bucharest, Romania
Ms Judy Turner-Crowson	Former Chair, World Association for Psychosocial Rehabilitation, WAPR Advocacy Committee, Hamburg, Germany
Mrs Pascale Van den Heede	Mental Health Europe, Brussels, Belgium
Ms Marianna Várfalvi-Bognarne	Ministry of Health, Hungary
Dr Uldis Veits	Riga Municipal Health Commission, Riga, Latvia
Mr Luc Vigneault	Association des Groupes de Défense des Droits en Santé Mentale du Québec, Canada
Dr Liwei Wang	Consultant, Ministry of Health, Beijing, People's Republic of China
Dr Xiangdong Wang	Acting Regional Adviser for Mental Health, WHO Regional Office for the Western Pacific, Manila, Philippines
Professor Harvey Whiteford	Department of Psychiatry, University of Queensland, Toowing Qld, Australia
Dr Ray G. Xerri	Department of Health, Floriana, Malta
Dr Xie Bin	Consultant, Ministry of Health, Beijing, People's Republic of China
Dr Xin Yu	Consultant, Ministry of Health, Beijing, People's Republic of China
Professor Shen Yucun	Institute of Mental Health, Beijing Medical University, People's Republic of China

Dr Taintor Zebulon	President, WAPR, Department of Psychiatry, New York University Medical Center, New York, USA

WHO also wishes to acknowledge the generous financial support of the Governments of Australia, Finland, Italy, the Netherlands, New Zealand, and Norway, as well as the Eli Lilly and Company Foundation and the Johnson and Johnson Corporate Social Responsibility, Europe.

"Mental health care should be provided through general health services and community settings. Large and centralized psychiatric institutions need to be replaced by other more appropriate mental health services."

Table of Contents

Preface

This module is part of the WHO Mental Health Policy and Service guidance package, which provides practical information to assist countries to improve the mental health of their populations.

What is the purpose of the guidance package?

The purpose of the guidance package is to assist policy-makers and planners to:

- develop policies and comprehensive strategies for improving the mental health of populations;
- use existing resources to achieve the greatest possible benefits;
- provide effective services to those in need;
- assist the reintegration of persons with mental disorders into all aspects of community life, thus improving their overall quality of life.

What is in the package?

The package consists of a series of interrelated user-friendly modules that are designed to address the wide variety of needs and priorities in policy development and service planning. The topic of each module represents a core aspect of mental health. The starting point is the module entitled The Mental Health Context, which outlines the global context of mental health and summarizes the content of all the modules. This module should give readers an understanding of the global context of mental health, and should enable them to select specific modules that will be useful to them in their own situations. Mental Health Policy, Plans and Programmes is a central module, providing detailed information about the process of developing policy and implementing it through plans and programmes. Following a reading of this module, countries may wish to focus on specific aspects of mental health covered in other modules.

The guidance package includes the following modules:

> The Mental Health Context
> Mental Health Policy, Plans and Programmes
> Mental Health Financing
> Mental Health Legislation and Human Rights
> Advocacy for Mental Health
> Organization of Services for Mental Health
> Quality Improvement for Mental Health
> Planning and Budgeting to Deliver Services for Mental Health

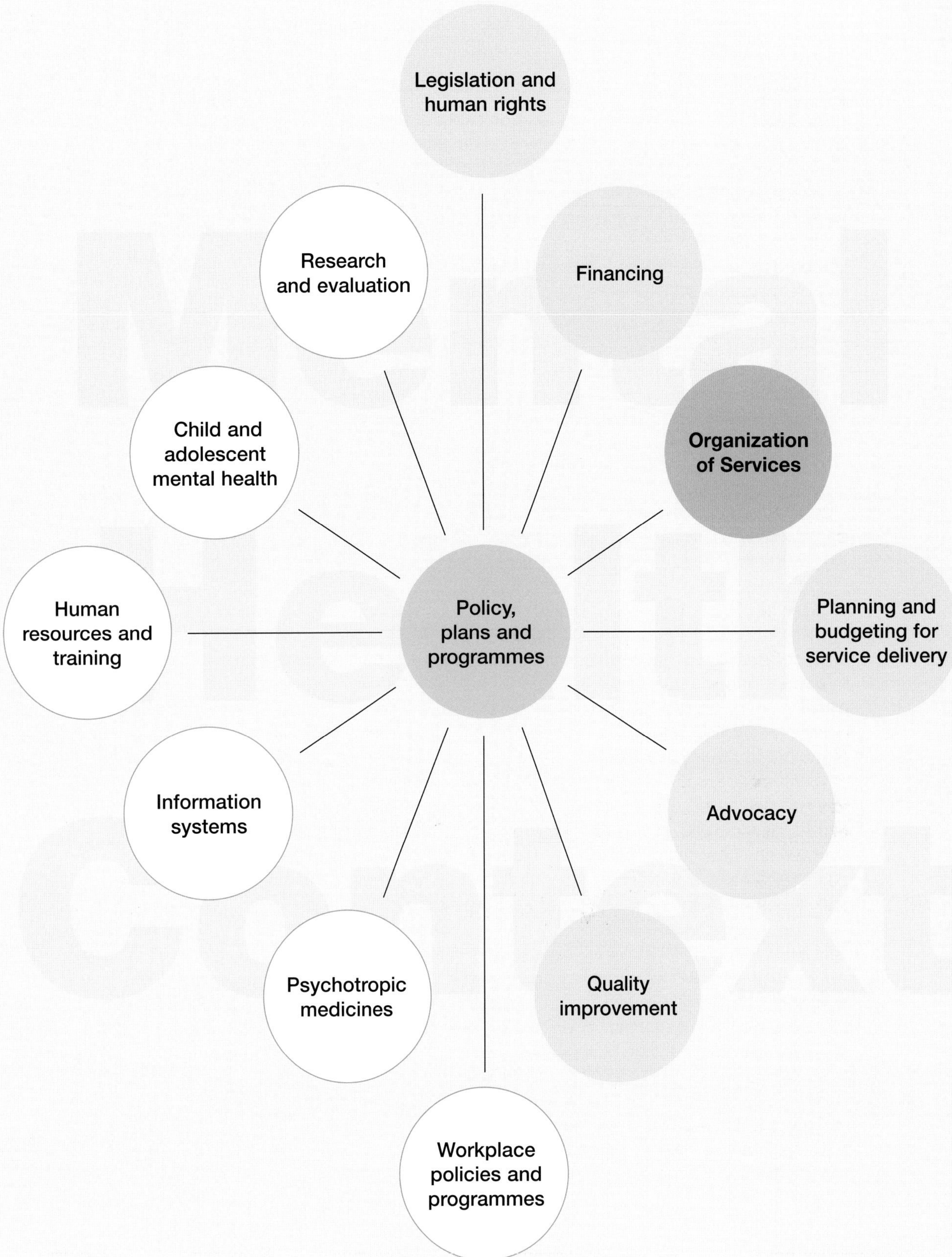

still to be developed

The following modules are not yet available but will be included in the final guidance package:

> Improving Access and Use of Psychotropic Medicines
> Mental Health Information Systems
> Human Resources and Training for Mental Health
> Child and Adolescent Mental Health
> Research and Evaluation of Mental Health Policy and Services
> Workplace Mental Health Policies and Programmes

Who is the guidance package for?

The modules will be of interest to:

- policy-makers and health planners;
- government departments at federal, state/regional and local levels;
- mental health professionals;
- groups representing people with mental disorders;
- representatives or associations of families and carers of people with mental disorders;
- advocacy organizations representing the interests of people with mental disorders and their relatives and families;
- nongovernmental organizations involved or interested in the provision of mental health services.

How to use the modules

- They can be used **individually or as a package**. They are cross-referenced with each other for ease of use. Countries may wish to go through each of the modules systematically or may use a specific module when the emphasis is on a particular area of mental health. For example, countries wishing to address mental health legislation may find the module entitled Mental Health Legislation and Human Rights useful for this purpose.

- They can be used as a **training package** for mental health policy-makers, planners and others involved in organizing, delivering and funding mental health services. They can be used as educational materials in university or college courses. Professional organizations may choose to use the package as an aid to training for persons working in mental health.

- They can be used as a framework for **technical consultancy** by a wide range of international and national organizations that provide support to countries wishing to reform their mental health policy and/or services.

- They can be used as **advocacy tools** by consumer, family and advocacy organizations. The modules contain useful information for public education and for increasing awareness among politicians, opinion-makers, other health professionals and the general public about mental disorders and mental health services.

Format of the modules

Each module clearly outlines its aims and the target audience for which it is intended. The modules are presented in a step-by-step format so as to assist countries in using and implementing the guidance provided. The guidance is not intended to be prescriptive or to be interpreted in a rigid way: countries are encouraged to adapt the material in accordance with their own needs and circumstances. Practical examples are given throughout.

There is extensive cross-referencing between the modules. Readers of one module may need to consult another (as indicated in the text) should they wish further guidance.

All the modules should be read in the light of WHO's policy of providing most mental health care through general health services and community settings. Mental health is necessarily an intersectoral issue involving the education, employment, housing, social services and criminal justice sectors. It is important to engage in serious consultation with consumer and family organizations in the development of policy and the delivery of services.

Dr Michelle Funk

Dr Benedetto Saraceno

ORGANIZATION OF SERVICES FOR MENTAL HEALTH

Introduction

Mental health services are the means by which effective interventions for mental health are delivered. The way these services are organized has an important bearing on their effectiveness and ultimately on whether they meet the aims and objectives of a mental health policy.

This module does not attempt to prescribe a single model for organizing services in a global context. The exact form of service organization and delivery ultimately depends on a country's social, cultural, political and economic context. However, research findings and experience in countries in different regions of the world point towards some of the key ingredients of successful service delivery models. This module indicates these ingredients in order to give countries guidance on the organization of their mental health services.

Description and analysis of mental health services around the world

The various components of mental health services are categorized below. This is not a recommendation on the organization of services but an attempt to broadly map the services that exist.

I) Mental health services integrated into the general health system can be as broadly grouped as those in primary care and those in general hospitals.

Mental health services in primary care include treatment services and preventive and promotional activities delivered by primary care professionals. Among them, for example, are services provided by general practitioners, nurses and other health staff based in primary care clinics. The provision of mental health care through primary care requires significant investment in training primary care professionals to detect and treat mental disorders. Such training should address the specific needs of different groups of primary care professionals such as doctors, nurses and community health workers. Furthermore, primary care staff should have the time to conduct mental health interventions. It may be necessary to increase the number of general health care staff if an additional mental health care component is to be provided through primary care.

For most common and acute mental disorders these services may have clinical outcomes that are as good as or better than those of more specialized mental health services. However, clinical outcomes are highly dependent on the quality of the services provided, which in turn depends on the knowledge of primary care staff and their skills in diagnosing and treating common mental disorders, as well as on the availability of drugs and other options for psychosocial treatment. Primary care services are easily accessible and are generally better accepted than other forms of service delivery by persons with mental health disorders. This is mainly attributable to the reduced stigma associated with seeking help from such services. Both providers and users generally find these services inexpensive in comparison with other mental health services.

Mental health services in general hospitals include certain services offered in district general hospitals and academic or central hospitals that form part of the general health system. Such services include psychiatric inpatient wards, psychiatric beds in general wards and emergency departments, and outpatient clinics. There may also be some specialist services, e.g. for children, adolescents and the elderly. These services are provided by specialist mental health professionals such as psychiatrists, psychiatric nurses, psychiatric social workers, psychologists, and physicians who have received special training in psychiatry. Clearly, such services require adequate numbers of trained specialist staff and adequate training facilities for them.

The clinical outcomes associated with these services are variable and depend on their quality and quantity. In many countries, the mental health services of general hospitals can manage acute behavioural emergencies and episodic disorders which require only outpatient treatment. However, their ability to help people with severe mental disorders depends on the availability of comprehensive primary care services or community mental health services and on the continuity of care that these provide. Mental health services based in general hospitals are usually well accepted. Because general hospitals are usually located in large urban centres, however, there may be problems of accessibility in countries lacking good transport systems. For service providers, mental health services in general hospitals are likely to be more expensive than services provided in primary care but less expensive than those provided in specialized institutions. Service users also have to incur additional travel and time costs that can create additional access barriers in some countries.

II) Community mental health services can be categorized as formal and informal.

Formal community mental health services include community-based rehabilitation services, hospital diversion programmes, mobile crisis teams, therapeutic and residential supervised services, home help and support services, and community-based services for special populations such as trauma victims, children, adolescents and the elderly. Community mental health services are not based in hospital settings but need close working links with general hospitals and mental hospitals. They work best if closely linked with primary care services and informal care providers working in the community. These services require some staff with a high level of skills and training, although many functions can be delivered by general health workers with some training in mental health. In many developing countries, highly skilled personnel of this kind are not readily available and this restricts the availability of such services to a small minority of people.

Well-resourced and well-funded community mental health services provide an opportunity for many persons with severe mental disorders to continue living in the community and thus promote community integration. High levels of satisfaction with community mental health services are associated with their accessibility, a reduced level of stigma associated with help-seeking for mental disorders and a reduced likelihood of violations of human rights. Community mental health services of good quality, providing a wide range of services to meet diverse clinical needs, are demanding in terms of cost and personnel. Reductions in costs relative to those of mental hospitals are likely to take many years to materialize.

Informal community mental health services may be provided by local community members other than general health professionals or dedicated mental health professionals and paraprofessionals. Informal providers are unlikely to form the core of mental health service provision and countries would be ill-advised to depend solely on their services, which, however, are a useful complement to formal mental health services and can be important in improving the outcomes of persons with mental disorders. Such service providers usually have high acceptability and there are few access barriers as the providers are nearly always based in the communities they serve. Although the services are classed as informal, not all of them are totally free. In many countries, for instance, traditional healers charge for their services and could therefore be considered as providing private formal health care services. Moreover, there are concerns about violations of human rights in relation to the treatment methods employed by some traditional healers and faith healers.

III) Institutional mental health services include specialist institutional services and mental hospitals. A key feature of these services is the independent stand-alone service style, although they may have some links with the rest of the health care system.

Specialist institutional mental health services are provided by certain outpatient clinics and by certain public or private hospital-based facilities that offer various services in inpatient wards. Among the services are those provided by acute and high security units, units for children and elderly people, and forensic psychiatry units. These services are not merely those of modernized mental hospitals: they meet very specific needs that require institutional settings and a large complement of specialist staff who have been properly trained. The scarcity of such staff presents a serious problem in developing countries. Specialist services are usually tertiary referral centres and patients who are difficult to treat make up a large proportion of their case-loads. If well funded and well resourced they provide care of high quality and produce outcomes that are good enough to justify their continuation. Nearly all specialist services have problems of access, both in developing countries and in the developed world. These problems may be associated with a lack of availability, with location in urban centres that have inadequate transport links, and with stigma attached to seeking help from such services. Specialist services are costly to set up and maintain, mainly because of the high level of investment in infrastructure and staff. In many developing countries the cost of specialist units is not necessarily high because staff costs are lower than in developed countries and, in many cases, investments are at a low level and units function in substandard conditions.

Dedicated mental hospitals mainly provide long-stay custodial services. In many parts of the world they are either the only mental health services or remain a substantial component of such services. In many countries they consume most of the available human and financial resources for mental health. This is a serious barrier to the development of alternative community-based mental health services. Mental hospitals are frequently associated with poor outcomes attributable to a combination of factors such as poor clinical care, violations of human rights, the nature of institutionalized care and a lack of rehabilitative activities. They therefore represent the least desirable use of scarce financial resources available for mental health services. This is particularly true in those developing countries where mental hospitals provide the only mental health services. Stigma associated with mental hospitals also reduces their acceptability and accessibility.

Current status of service organization around the world

Very few countries have an optimal mix of services. Some developing countries made mental health services more widely available by integrating them into primary care services. Other countries have also made mental health services available at general hospitals. In some countries there are good examples of intersectoral collaboration between non-governmental organizations, academic institutions, public sector health services, informal mental health services and users, leading to the development of community-based services. Even within countries there are usually significant disparities between different regions, and both types of service are only available to small proportions of populations, usually in urban areas or selected rural areas.

In developed countries the process of deinstitutionalization during the last three decades has led to reductions in the populations of mental hospitals and to the closure of many of these institutions. However, this has not been accompanied by sufficient provision of community-based services, which are often inadequate and unevenly distributed. There is insufficient emphasis on developing mental health services in primary care. For example, although depression is a common problem in primary care settings, it is still not identified or is undertreated by primary care practitioners in many developed countries.

Two main conclusions can be drawn from global experience. Firstly, mental health services pose challenges in both developing countries and developed countries. However, the nature of the challenges differs. In many developing countries there is gross underprovision of resources, personnel and services, and these matters need immediate attention. In developed countries some of the problems relate to insufficient community reprovision, the need to promote the detection and treatment of mental disorders in primary care settings, and the competing demands of general psychiatric services and specialist services. Secondly, more expensive specialist services are not the answer to these problems. Even within the resource constraints of health services in most countries, significant improvements in delivery are possible by redirecting resources towards services that are less expensive, have reasonably good oucomes and benefit increased proportions of populations.

Guidance for organizing services

The recommendations in this module are intended to form an integrated system of service delivery and should not be interpreted in isolation from each other. None of the recommendations can be expected to succeed on its own in improving the care of persons with mental disorders. Service organization should be based on principles of accessibility, coordinated care, continuity of care, effectiveness, equity and respect for human rights.

Service planners have to determine the exact mix of different types of mental health services and the level of provision of particular service delivery channels. The absolute requirement for various services differs greatly between countries but the relative needs of different services are broadly similar in many countries. It is clear that the most numerous services should be informal community mental health services and community-based mental health services provided by primary care staff, followed by psychiatric services based in general hospitals, formal community mental health services and, lastly, specialist mental health services. There is little justification for including the kind of services provided by mental hospitals. There will always be a need for long-stay facilities for an extremely small proportion of patients, even if the provision of community-based services is of a high order. However, most of these patients can be accommodated in small units located in the community, approximating community living as far as possible, or alternatively, in small long-stay wards in hospitals that also provide other specialist services. Custodial care in large institutions, as provided by mental hospitals, is not justified by its cost, its effectiveness or the quality of care provided.

The integration of mental health services into general health services helps to reduce the stigma associated with seeking help from stand-alone mental health services. It also helps to overcome the acute shortage of mental health professionals and to encourage the early identification of mental disorders in people presenting with psychosomatic symptoms in general health services. Other potential benefits include possibilities for providing care in the community and opportunities for community involvement in care. The integration of mental health services into general health services is the most viable strategy for extending mental health services to underserved populations.

Integration can be pursued at the clinical, managerial, administrative and financial levels. Potentially, however, full integration has both benefits and drawbacks, and countries have to take their own circumstances into account when choosing between full and partial integration. There should be good integration at least at the clinical level. This involves integration into primary care settings, the integration of mental health services into general hospitals, the development of links between primary care and secondary services and the integration of mental health into other established health and social programmes.

Integration into primary care requires that primary care staff be trained to assume responsibilities for the provision of mental health services and the promotion of mental health. Many countries also need to invest in additional primary care staff so that they have sufficient time to deliver mental health interventions. Among other issues that need to be addressed are the provision of adequate infrastructures, the availability of equipment and, most importantly, the availability of psychotropic medication.

Integration into general hospitals requires the provision of facilities such as outpatient departments and psychiatric wards in general hospitals as well as the availability of mental health professionals, e.g. psychiatrists, psychologists, psychiatric nurses and social workers.

The need for good linkages between primary health care and secondary mental health facilities cannot be overstressed. A clear referral and linkage system should be put in place and operated in consultation with service providers at the district and regional levels.

In developing countries the integration of mental health services into established physical health and social programmes provides a feasible and affordable way of implementing mental health programmes. Thus maternal depression can be tackled as within a wider reproductive health programme, women's mental health can be considered in programmes concerned with domestic violence, and mental health needs can be dealt with in HIV/AIDS programmes.

It is necessary for countries to build formal and informal mental health services. The development of community services is essential if dependence on institutional services is to be reduced. In developing countries the lack of financial and human resources requires these services to be developed in a phased manner that varies with local priorities for specific community services. Developing countries also have to utilize existing networks of nongovernmental organizations for providing some of these community-based services, e.g. clubhouses, support groups, employment or rehabilitation workshops, sheltered workshops, supervised work placements, and staffed residential accommodation.

Deinstitutionalization is an essential part of the reform of mental health services. This means more than discharging people from long-stay hospitals. It requires significant changes involving the use of community-based alternatives rather than institutions for the delivery of services. The provision of services in the community should go hand-in-hand with reducing the populations of mental hospitals. Deinstitutionalization can proceed in stages once community-based alternatives are in place. Achieving it requires strong commitment among planners, managers and clinicians.

Key issues in the organization of mental health services

The above recommendations for organizing mental health services should take into account the evidence base for mental health interventions, the unique needs of those with mental disorders, the way communities and patients access services and other important structural issues such as the need for intersectoral collaboration.

There is evidence that community-based treatment is associated with substantially better outcomes than inpatient treatment and care, and that shorter stays in hospital are as effective as longer stays. Some conditions, e.g. depression, can be effectively treated by primary care personnel using a combination of medications and counselling or psychotherapy. With regard to schizophrenia, regular medication and family intervention can substantially reduce the relapse rate and thus improve patients' quality of life.

Health care systems should orient themselves towards the needs of the many persons with severe and long-term mental disorders. These people are ill-served by a throughput model of care that emphasizes the importance of vigorous treatment of acute episodes in the expectation that most patients will make a reasonably complete recovery without the need for continuing care until the next acute episode. A continuing care approach is more appropriate for people with severe and long-term mental disorders. It emphasizes the need to address the totality of patients' needs, including social, occupational and psychological requirements.

The pathways to care, i.e. the routes whereby people with mental disorders access the providers of mental health services, differ between developed and developing countries because of different levels of health system development. These pathways may occasionally hinder access to mental health services, resulting in delays in help-seeking and a higher likelihood of poor long-term outcomes. Planners should design service delivery so as to overcome the barriers, improve access and thus reduce the duration and severity of disability caused by mental disorders.

Planners should aim to eliminate disparities in mental health services between rural and urban settings. Examples are given in the present module of programmes that attempt to diminish such disparities.

Services are usually organized from a managerial perspective and users are forced to adjust to the particular structure of the service they wish to access. This service-led approach is characteristic of many mental health services. Unlike the needs-led approach, it results in significant barriers to access, especially for people with severe mental disorders whose needs go beyond purely medical and therapeutic interventions. There is a move towards models of service provision that are needs-led, e.g. case management, assertive treatment programmes and psychiatric rehabilitation villages in rural areas. These models are an acknowledgment that the needs of patients should be placed first and that services should adapt their organization to meet these needs.

The complex needs of many persons with mental disorders cannot be met by the health sector alone. Intersectoral collaboration is therefore essential. Collaboration is needed both within the health sector (intrasectoral collaboration) and outside the health sector (intersectoral collaboration).

Acknowledging the need for collaborative efforts is the first step towards enhancing collaboration between and within sectors. Mental health agencies and persons involved in the planning and delivery of mental health services should take a lead in explaining what is required to other people, especially people outside the health sector. Collaboration can be improved by involving other sectors in policy formulation, delegating the responsibility for certain activities to agencies from other sectors, establishing information networks with agencies from other sectors and among other measures, by establishing a national advisory committee with the participation of relevant agencies from sectors outside mental health.

The last two sections in this module present recommendations for immediate action, discuss barriers to the implementation of services and outline possible ways of overcoming them.

Aims and target audience

This module aims to:

- present a description and analysis of mental health services around the world, examining different services and their organization and activities;
- review the current status of service organization around the world;
- make recommendations for organizing services;
- discuss crucial issues in the organization of services;
- discuss barriers to the organization of services and suggest solutions.

The module will be of interest to:

- policy-makers and health planners;
- government departments at the national, regional and local levels;
- mental health professionals;
- people with mental disorders and their representative organizations;
- representatives or associations of families and carers of persons with mental disorders;
- advocacy organizations representing the interests of persons with mental disorders and their relatives and families;
- nongovernmental organizations involved or interested in the provision of mental health services.

1. Introduction

Services are the means by which effective interventions for mental health are delivered. The organization of services is therefore a critical aspect of mental health care. At best, the way in which mental health services are organized enhances the aims and objectives of national mental health policy. Poorly organized services fail to meet the expectations and needs of people with mental disorders and impose costs without commensurate benefits.

The organization of services is a critical aspect of mental health care.

This module does not attempt to prescribe a single model for the organization of services in a global context. The exact form of service organization and delivery depends on the social, cultural, political and economic context. The availability of financial and human resources differs between countries. Cultural aspirations and values also differ, even between different regions in particular countries. Consequently, it is highly unlikely that any given model of service delivery can fully meet the needs of all persons with mental disorders in all countries.

The exact form of service organization and delivery depends on the local context.

However, practical experience in countries and research findings in different regions of the world point towards certain **key ingredients** of successful models of service delivery. The present module sets out these key ingredients in order to provide guidance to countries on the organization of their mental health services. It is aimed at all countries interested in restructuring their mental health services.

In spite of global diversity, certain key ingredients of successful service organization can be identified.

2. Description and analysis of mental health services around the world

A schematic representation of different components of mental health services found across the world is given in Figure 1. The framework aims to broadly map the variety of services in different countries with varying health systems and varying levels of care provision. It is not a recommendation on organization but an attempt to describe various types of services.

Figure 1: Components of mental health services

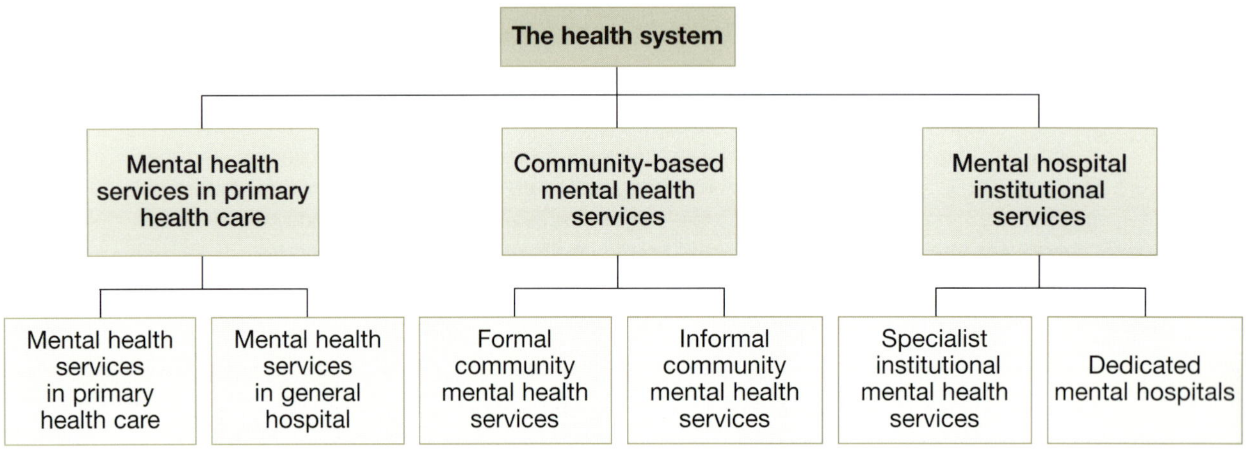

Each of the categories is described in detail below. The descriptions are followed by brief discussions of the implications, potential benefits and disadvantages of each category for service providers and people with mental disorders.

2.1 Mental health services integrated into the general health system

Two service categories can be identified within the broad category of integrated mental health services:

- mental health services in primary care;
- mental health services in general hospitals.

2.1.1 Mental health services in primary care

This category includes treatment and preventive and promotional interventions conducted by primary care professionals. Examples are given below. Of course, all of these interventions do not necessarily take place in every country. Furthermore, specialist staff rather than primary care professionals may perform some of the functions described in the examples below. The way in which countries organize these activities may vary, depending on the context, e.g. the organization of services and the availability of specialist staff.

Primary care services may include mental health care and promotional and preventive activities conducted by primary care professionals.

Following are some examples of primary care providers:

a) general practitioners, nurses and other health care staff based in primary care clinics providing diagnostic, treatment and referral services for mental disorders;
b) general practitioners, nurses and other workers making home visits for the management of mental disorders;
c) non-medical primary care staff providing basic health services in rural areas;
d) non-medical primary care staff involved in health promotion and prevention activities, e.g. running clinics for mental health education and screening for mental disorders in schools;
e) primary care workers and aid workers providing information, education, guidance and treatment interventions for trauma victims in the context of natural disasters and acts of violence.

Potential benefits and disadvantages of primary care services

I) Human resources: Providing mental health care through primary care requires significant investment in training primary care professionals to detect and treat mental disorders. Such training should address the specific practical training needs of different groups of primary care professionals, e.g. doctors, nurses and community health workers. Preferably, ongoing training programmes should be provided rather than single workshops that do not provide subsequent support for reinforcing new skills. In many countries this has not happened and primary health care professionals are not well equipped to work with people who have mental disorders and who therefore receive suboptimal care. Primary care staff are generally well qualified to provide help for people with physical disorders but many are uncomfortable about dealing with mental disorders. Indeed, many primary care staff may question their role in managing mental disorders. Training programmes should include coverage of these issues.

Significant investment is needed in the training of primary care professionals.

A related issue is that one of the main reasons for the reluctance of some primary care staff to provide mental health services is that they do not have sufficient time to conduct the required interventions. It may be necessary to increase the number of primary care staff if they are to add mental health care to their practice. However, it has been argued that primary care workers can save time by addressing the mental health needs of people who present to services with physical complaints that have a psychological etiology (Goldberg & Lecrubier, 1995; Üstün and Sartorius, 1995).

Increased numbers of primary care professionals may be needed to deliver mental health interventions

II) Clinical outcomes: Conventional logic suggests that basic primary services yield less favourable outcomes than more specialized services but this is not necessarily true. For most common and acute mental disorders these services may give equally good or superior clinical outcomes (see Section 7.1). There are three possible explanations for this. First, users are more likely to seek early help for mental disorders because of reduced costs and high acceptability. Second, there is an opportunity for the early detection of mental disorders when users seek help for physical problems. Third, primary care workers may have a greater insight than more specialized workers into the cultural

For a number of mental disorders, good clinical outcomes can be obtained in primary care settings .

and interpersonal contexts of service users. Users may thus feel more understood at the primary care level. Moreover, service providers may recognize strengths in users' cultural and interpersonal contexts which can be exploited for therapeutic purposes. However, clinical outcomes are highly dependent on the quality of the services provided, as affected by the knowledge of primary care staff, their skills in diagnosing and treating common mental disorders, the time available, and access to psychotropic medication and psychosocial treatment.

III) Acceptability: Primary health care services are generally relatively acceptable to people with mental disorders. Less stigma is associated with seeking help from primary care services, partly because they provide both physical and mental health care. Furthermore, primary care services are less likely to result in violations of the human rights of persons with mental disorders.

Primary care services are well accepted.

IV) Access: Access to primary care services is good as they are geographically close to users and are usually open at times determined with reference to local work patterns. Access is also favoured by comparatively low indirect costs. These increase the probability of poor people using such services.

Primary care services are generally more accessible.

V) Financial costs: These services tend to be less expensive than others because of lower human resource costs, reduced costs of physical facilities as a result of the joint use of facilities for general health care, less need for specialized equipment and less use of inpatient facilities. There are lower indirect costs for people with mental disorders because these services tend to be geographically closer to the patients so that less travelling and time are required in order to benefit from them.

Mental health interventic delivered through prima care may be less expens than other forms of service delivery.

2.1.2 Mental health services in general hospitals

A number of mental health services may be offered in secondary district or tertiary academic/central hospitals that form part of the general health system. Common facilities for adults include psychiatric inpatient wards, psychiatric beds in general wards, psychiatric emergency departments and outpatient clinics. Services for children and adolescents are found in general, academic or children's hospitals. These may include psychiatric wards for children and adolescents and child/adolescent outpatient clinics. Services for the elderly are found in general and academic hospitals and include psychogeriatric wards, psychiatric beds in other wards, and outpatient clinics. These services are provided by specialist mental health professionals such as psychiatrists, psychiatric nurses, psychiatric social workers, psychologists, and physicians with special training in psychiatry. Examples of mental health services offered by general hospitals are given in Box 1.

Certain mental health services may be provide in district general hospit and in tertiary and academic hospitals.

Box 1. Mental health services offered by general hospitals

- Acute inpatient care
- Crisis stabilization care
- Partial (day/night) hospital programmes
- Consultation/liaison services for general medical patients
- Intensive/planned outpatient programmes
- Respite care
- Expert consultation/support/training for primary care services
- Multidisciplinary psychiatric teams linked with other local and provincial sectors (schools, employers, correctional services, welfare) and nongovernmental organizations in intersectoral prevention and promotion initiatives
- Specialized units/wards for persons with specific mental disorders and for related rehabilitation programmes

Potential benefits and disadvantages of mental health services in general hospitals

I) Human resources: These services require adequate numbers of specialist mental health professionals such as psychiatrists, psychologists, psychiatric social workers and psychiatric nurses. Consequently, investment is necessary in facilities where such staff can be trained. There are a number of advantages in having mental health professionals who are based in general hospitals. They can participate in undergraduate and postgraduate medical teaching and training, thus sensitizing physicians to mental disorders. Psychiatric departments in general hospitals can act as centres for postgraduate training in psychiatry and can provide opportunities for training other mental health professionals, e.g. psychologists, nurses and social workers.

Specialist human resources are needed for mental health in general hospitals.

II) Clinical outcomes: These vary, depending on the quality and quantity of the services provided. In many developing countries the only mental health services in general hospitals are outpatient departments, short-stay inpatient wards for the acutely ill, and consultation/liaison services provided by psychiatric departments to other medical departments. In such circumstances, mental health services can manage acute behavioural emergencies reasonably well but have little to offer persons with severe mental disorders who may enter an admission-discharge-readmission cycle (the revolving door syndrome) unless comprehensive primary care services or community services are also available. The absence of psychotherapy and psychosocial therapies also limits the ability of such services to improve outcomes for people suffering from non-psychotic illnesses.

Clinical outcomes depend on the quality and quantity of service provision.

III) Acceptability: General hospital-based services are usually acceptable to people with mental disorders. There is less stigma associated with obtaining help from such services than from dedicated mental hospitals. The open nature of general hospitals makes it less likely that violations of human rights will occur than in closed institutions.

These services are generally acceptable to people with mental disorders.

IV) Access: General hospital services are usually located in district headquarters while tertiary/academic centres are usually located in big cities. Particularly in developing countries, access to services based in general hospitals can be hindered by the financial costs. The lack of reliable and cheap public transport services in many countries may exclude many people who do not live in the urban areas where such hospitals are sited. However, mental health services based in general hospitals have the advantages of relatively easy access to specialist investigations and treatment as well as medical treatment for comorbid physical illnesses.

Mental health services based in general hospitals have some access problems but also enjoy certain advantages.

V) Financial costs: For service providers, mental health services in general hospitals are likely to be more costly than services provided in primary care settings. This is because of infrastructural costs, the costs of providing for inpatient care, and higher staff costs attributable to the use of specialist personnel such as psychiatrists and other mental health professionals. However, mental health services in general hospitals may be less expensive than services provided in specialized institutions. For users, services based in general hospitals tend to cost more than those based in primary care settings because of the additional costs of travelling and the loss of employment, i.e. indirect costs. In rural areas, general hospital-based services save transport costs for service providers by transferring them to users. This transfer of financial burden can create access barriers in developing countries, in many of which the indirect costs are disproportionately high in comparison with people's ability to spend directly on mental health services.

These services are more expensive to provide tha those in primary care se but may be less expensi than services provided i specialist institutions.

2.2 Community mental health services

Community mental health services can be subdivided into those that are formal and those that are informal.

2.2.1 Formal community mental health services

Formal community mental health services include a wide array of settings and different levels of care provided by mental health professionals and paraprofessionals, i.e. people who work alongside professionals in an auxiliary capacity. These services include community-based rehabilitation services, hospital diversion programmes, mobile crisis teams, therapeutic and residential supervised services, home help and support services, and community-based services for special populations such as trauma victims, children, adolescents and the elderly. Community mental health services are not based in hospital settings but need close working links with general hospitals and mental hospitals. These links may include, for example, a two-way referral system whereby general hospitals and mental hospitals accept patients for short-term management and refer patients who are to be discharged into the community. Community mental health services work best when they are closely linked with primary care services and informal care providers working in the community. Box 2 gives examples of formal community mental health services.

Community mental healt services need good links with primary and second health care and also with providers of informal community mental health services.

Box 2. **Examples of formal community mental health services**

Rehabilitation services

- Community mental health centres/outpatient clinics
- Clubhouses
- Day care centres
- Drop-in centres
- Support groups
- Employment/rehabilitation workshops
- Sheltered workshops
- Supervised work placements
- Cooperative work schemes
- Supported employment programmes

Hospital diversion programmes and mobile crisis teams

- Mobile services for crisis assessment and treatment (including evenings and weekends) operating from community mental health centres or outpatient clinics

Crisis services

- Ordinary houses in neighbourhood settings with 24-hour care given by mental health professionals
- Support staff with mental health training and knowledge who can stay in a patient's own home overnight to provide support and supervision during a period of crisis
- Crisis centres

Therapeutic and supervised residential services

- Apartment buildings for ex-patients (unsupervised)
- Scattered apartments each occupied by two or three residents (unsupervised)
- Group homes (staffed and unstaffed)
- Hostels
- Halfway houses
- Psychiatric agricultural rehabilitation villages
- Ordinary housing

Home health services

- Assessment, treatment and management coordinated by a home care clinician from a community mental health centre
- Case management and assertive community treatment
- Domiciliary support centres

Others

- Clinical services in educational, employment and correctional settings
- Telephone hotline services
- Trauma relief programmes in refugee camps or community settings

I) Human resources: Formal community mental health services require at least some staff with a high level of skills and training. However, many functions can be delivered by health workers with some training in mental health. The labour-intensive nature of community mental health services means that greater numbers of staff are needed than in other mental health services in order to maximize reach.

Community mental healt services require speciali staff in adequate numbe This may be difficult to achieve in developing countries.

II) Clinical outcomes: These depend on the quality of service provision. Well-resourced and well-funded community mental health services give many people who have severe mental disorders an opportunity to continue living in the community, thus promoting community integration (see Section 7.1). Many community mental health services, e.g. day centres, sheltered workshops and supported housing, play a crucial role in giving social care to people with mental disorders. This can have a significantly positive impact on clinical outcomes and the quality of life.

Well-resourced services have reasonably good outcomes.

III) Acceptability: High levels of satisfaction with community mental health services are associated with their accessibility, reduced stigma associated with help-seeking for mental disorders and a reduced likelihood of human rights violations.

These services generally enjoy high levels of user satisfaction.

IV) Access: Community mental health services are highly accessible to users, especially those with severe mental disorders requiring continuing input from mental health services. These services are less stigmatizing than segregated mental hospitals, and this further improves their accessibility. The main barriers to access arise from the paucity of such services, which may be attributable to the high costs of setting up and running them and to shortages of trained personnel. These barriers are especially noticeable in developing countries, where community mental health services are usually only available to a small minority of people. Rural populations and minorities in developed countries face similar barriers to access because of the unavailability of such services.

Community mental health services are highl accessible to users.

V) Financial costs: In many countries, deinstitutionalization followed by community reprovision has been driven by the expectation of lower costs for service providers, especially public health providers. However, experience during the past decade suggests that the cost savings are minimal, particularly in the short term. Community service providers have to incur additional expenditure on travel and transport for staff, especially in rural areas. Additionally, fewer users can be assisted because of the time required for travelling. Community mental health services of good quality which provide a wide range of services meeting diverse clinical needs are cost-intensive and personnel-intensive. Any cost savings are likely to take many years to materialize. Savings result from reduced use of inpatient beds, which are an expensive resource in most developed countries and many developing countries. There are cost savings for people with mental disorders through reduced travel and reduced indirect costs as services go to the user rather than the other way round.

Community services are not inexpensive and do not necessarily result in overall cost savings for service providers.

2.2.2 Informal community mental health services

In addition to professionals and paraprofessionals in the fields of general health or mental health, local community members may provide a variety of mental health services. Although these people may have received little or no formal training in mental health skills, they can provide much of the required care, especially in settings where people with mental disorders live at home with their families. Informal mental health providers vary according to the different mental health resource scenarios and sociopolitical situations of countries and regions. Box 3 contains examples of providers of informal community mental health services.

Providers of informal community mental health services are unlikely to form the core of mental health service provision. Countries would be ill-advised to depend solely on these services. However, they are a useful complement to formal mental health services.

Informal providers cannot be solely relied on to provide mental health services.

Traditional healers do not easily fit into specific service categories in this section. Traditional healers may be faith healers, spiritual healers, religious healers or practitioners of indigenous or alternative systems of medicine. In some countries they may be part of the informal health sector. However, in many others they charge for their services and should therefore be considered as part of the privately provided formal health care services. In many countries they are the first point of contact for a majority of people with mental disorders and sometimes they give the only available services. They also have high acceptability and in general are readily accessible because they are usually members of the local communities that they serve. Notwithstanding the important role played by traditional healers in many societies in providing care to persons with mental disorders, it should be noted that some traditional healing practices have been associated with human rights violations. In particular there are concerns about violations of the rights of vulnerable groups, e.g. children, women and the elderly.

Traditional healers are a heterogeneous group.

Box 3. Examples of providers of informal community mental health services

- Traditional healers
- Village or community workers
- Family members
- Self-help and user groups
- Advocacy services
- Lay volunteers providing parental and youth education on mental health issues and screening for mental disorders (including suicidal tendencies) in clinics and schools
- Religious leaders providing health information on trauma reactions in complex emergencies
- Day care services provided by relatives, neighbours or retired members of local communities
- Humanitarian aid workers in complex emergencies.

Potential benefits and disadvantages of informal community mental health services

I) Human resources: In general these are readily obtainable in most communities, especially in rural and isolated communities where formal health services are not easily available.

Human resources are easily available in most communities.

II) Clinical outcomes: These services can play an important supportive role in improving outcomes for persons with mental disorders. They are important for maintaining integration in communities and providing support networks that minimize the risk of relapse. In many developing countries they are the main source of mental health provision and are most likely to be used by people with acute, brief and psychosocial stress-driven mental disorders.

Informal services can play an important role in supporting formal mental health services.

III) Acceptability: This tends to be high as communities perceive them as being more responsive to their expressed needs. These services are usually consonant with community perceptions and explanatory models of mental disorders and their treatment. There are, however, some concerns about human rights violations, especially regarding the use of traumatic treatment methods and the risk of violations of the rights of vulnerable populations, e.g. children, women and the elderly. Interventions are not subject to quality control measures such as may apply to public providers.

They usually have high acceptability in local communities.

IV) Access: There are few access barriers because these services are nearly always based in the community and enjoy a high degree of acceptability, thus reducing the likelihood of stigma associated with their use.

There are few access barriers.

V) Financial costs: Informal mental health services generally enjoy a significant cost advantage in comparison with nearly all formal mental health services (see discussion on traditional healers above). However, not all these services are necessarily free and users may have to bear some costs.

They are not always free and users may have to bear some costs.

2.3 Institutional services in mental hospitals

The key feature of these services is their independent stand-alone style, although they may have some links with the rest of the health care system. They can be subdivided into specialist institutional mental health services and dedicated mental hospitals.

2.3.1 Specialist institutional mental health services

These are usually specialist public or private hospital-based facilities offering various services in inpatient wards and in specialist outpatient clinic settings. They are not merely modernized mental hospitals but are services that attend to very specific needs requiring an institutional setting. Furthermore, they are not expected to provide primary mental health services to the general population but act as secondary and tertiary referral services. They include acute and high-security units, specialist units for children and elderly people, and other specialist services such as forensic psychiatry units. Examples of these services are given in Box 4.

Box 4. Examples of specialist institutional mental health services

> Specialist inpatient care
- Medium-security units
- High-security units

> Specialized units/centres for the treatment of specific disorders and for related rehabilitation programmes, e.g. eating disorder units

> Specialist clinics or units dedicated to specific mental disorders of children and adolescents

> Rehabilitation services for specific disorders of children and adolescents, e.g. autism and psychotic disorders

> Respite care

> Specialist clinics or units dedicated to specific disorders of the elderly, e.g. Alzheimer's disease

Potential benefits and disadvantages of specialist institutional services in mental hospitals

I) Human resources: Specialist services require a large complement of trained specialist mental health staff. Shortages of such staff are a serious problem in developing countries. The absence of trained personnel can make it difficult to maintain the desired quality of service and creates a risk of skewing the service towards custodial care with little therapeutic input.

Shortages of human resources affect the quality of specialist services.

II) Clinical outcomes: Specialist services are usually tertiary referral centres. Patients with mental disorders that are difficult to treat make up a large proportion of their case-loads. The success of specialist services is highly dependent on the quality of services and infrastructure available to them. In developed countries, where many of these specialist services are well funded and well resourced, they provide care of high quality with sufficiently good outcomes to justify their continuation. In developing countries the lack of finances, infrastructure and personnel usually means that many of these services are absent or inadequate.

Specialist services help many patients with severe mental disorders that are difficult to treat.

III) Acceptability: As with all segregated mental health institutions, specialist mental health services are associated with social stigma and consequently may not be highly acceptable. Service users are frequently reluctant to use these services except as a last resort. This may not necessarily be a problem as specialist services are not expected to encourage people to use them as first-line care providers.

Specialist services are not first-line care providers.

IV) Access: Nearly all specialist services have problems of access both in developed and developing countries. Many of these services are not easily available, even in developed countries, and are almost absent in developing countries. These specialist services are located in the vicinity of large urban areas but are frequently at some distance from them. Transport links to the hospitals in question may be inadequate, resulting in high costs of access. Stigma associated with segregated mental health services provided by specialist facilities acts as a barrier to use. Some of the access problems do not have easy answers. It is arguable, however, that specialist services should not be readily accessible services of first resort. For reasons of sustainability, moreover, specialist services have to be centralized and access has to be limited by the requirement of a professional referral.

Specialist services have some problems with geographical access.

V) Financial costs: The cost of setting up and running specialist services is high in comparison with that of other forms of service delivery. The reasons for this include the high level of investment required to set up dedicated units and the high staff costs associated with low ratios of staff to patients. In addition, costs rise because institutions have to care for individual patients over long periods of time. In many developing countries the cost of specialist units is not necessarily high because staff costs are lower than in developed countries, and investments are often at a low level as units function in substandard conditions. It is difficult to evaluate the financial disadvantage of specialist mental health services in such circumstances. However, if specialist services of good quality were provided in developing countries the above financial issues would apply equally to them. The exact distribution of these costs between service providers and service users depends on the funding arrangements in particular countries. Even when such services are publicly funded the users incur the indirect costs of obtaining care from them.

Specialist services of good quality are costly because of heavy invest in infrastructure and sta

2.3.2 Dedicated mental hospitals

These are old-style mental hospitals, mainly providing long-stay custodial services. In many parts of the world they provide either the only mental health services or a substantial component of such services. This may appear to contradict Atlas data indicating that only 37% of countries have no community care facilities, that 87% of countries have identified mental health as an activity in primary care, and that regular training of primary care personnel takes place in 59% of countries (World Health Organization, 2001b). However, these percentages do not reflect population coverage. Thus India, with a population in excess of 1 billion, has a community mental health programme in 22 districts covering a population of only 40 million (Jacob, 2001).

Potential benefits and disadvantages of mental hospitals

I) Human resources: In many countries, mental hospitals consume most of the available specialist mental health resources. This acts as a serious barrier to the development of alternative community-based mental health services. Moreover, there are high rates of staff burnout and demotivation and there is a gradual decline in skills of mental health professionals.

Mental hospitals consur a significant proportion financial and human resources in many coun

II) Clinical outcomes: Many of these institutions provide only custodial care of the kind found in prisons, frequently of extremely poor quality. Clinical outcomes are poor because of a combination of factors, e.g. poor clinical care, human rights violations, the nature of the institutionalized care process and a lack of rehabilitative activity. High costs and poor clinical outcomes mean that these institutions represent the least desirable use of the scarce financial resources available for mental health services. This is particularly true in developing countries where mental hospitals offer the only mental health services.

Clinical outcomes are pc because of the generally quality of service provid in many mental hospital

III) Acceptability: Mental hospitals generally do not enjoy high acceptability among people with mental disorders and communities. Significant stigma is associated with segregated mental hospitals, and people are usually reluctant to use these services except as a last resort. This results in delays in seeking treatment from such services, which in turn adversely affects clinical outcomes. Mental hospitals in developing and developed countries have a history of serious human rights violations. During the past two decades this has led to either their closure or their comprehensive reform. In spite of the improvements made, serious human rights concerns still surround the remaining long-stay mental hospitals in developed and developing countries.

Mental hospitals are ofte associated with stigma a human rights violations.

There is a reluctance to use these services.

IV) Access: Nearly all mental hospitals have problems related to access. They are usually based at some distance from urban areas and have poor transport links. People with mental disorders who are kept in these institutions may be isolated from their families because, for example, it is often very difficult to receive visitors or maintain contact with the outside world. Access is also hampered by cumbersome procedures related to admission and discharge and by the stigma associated with such institutions.

There are significant access barriers in most countries.

V) Financial costs: Mental hospitals are expensive and, in many developing countries, consume a significant portion of the budget meant for mental health services, leaving few resources for community-based initiatives. In Indonesia, for example, 97% of the mental health budget is spent on public mental hospitals (Trisnantoro, 2002). Many of the hospitals tend to be of a fixed nature with static long-stay populations of patients.

High financial costs leave few resources for alternative services.

Key points: Mental health services

- Mental health services can be broadly categorized as: (I) mental health services integrated into general health services; (II) community-based mental health services (III) institutional services provided by mental hospitals.

- Mental health services in primary care require significant investment in adequate human resources and appropriate training for primary care professionals.

- Good clinical outcomes for many mental disorders are possible through services delivered in primary care settings.

- Mental health services in primary care enjoy significant advantages of access, acceptability and lower financial costs for both providers and users.

- Mental health services in general hospitals require the presence of trained mental health professionals in sufficient numbers.

- Formal community mental health services need close working links with primary care and with secondary and tertiary hospital-based services.

- There is usually a high degree of satisfaction with well-resourced community services among users and their carers.

- The provision of community-based mental health services does not produce immediate cost savings for service providers.

- Providers of informal community mental health services are a readily available resource in many countries.

- Informal community mental health services are the first contact and sometimes the only providers in many developing countries.

- Specialist hospital-based services are needed in most countries although the absolute requirement for them differs between countries and is significantly lower than that for primary care and community-based mental health services.

- Dedicated mental hospitals are associated with stigma and human rights violations in many countries.

- In many countries, dedicated mental hospitals consume a disproportionate amount of financial and human resources, with the result that little scope is left for the development of alternative services.

3. Current status of service organization around the world

Very few countries have an optimal mix of services. Even within countries there are usually significant geographical disparities between regions.

Many countries rely on mental hospitals as the main providers of mental health care. These hospitals are usually located at a considerable distance from urban areas. This, along with poor transport facilities, emphasizes the segregation of people with mental disorders. The physical appearance of the hospitals is often menacing: many are surrounded by high walls with sentry towers, reflecting the custodial nature of the care provided. The institutions are often poorly equipped. Basic amenities such as toilets, beds and personal space for private belongings are often unavailable. Staff/patient ratios may be very low. This makes it unlikely that patients will receive professional attention of good quality on an individual basis. Human rights violations of all kinds are common. Box 5 contains an extract from a report of the National Human Rights Commission of India on the workings of the country's mental hospitals. It provides a good insight into the nature of such institutions and the difficulty of reforming them in order to overcome basic problems.

Human rights violations are still a significant problem in many mental hospitals in both developing and developed countries.

Box 5. Functioning of mental hospitals in India

The National Human Rights Commission of India investigated the 37 public mental hospitals in India housing nearly 18 000 patients. A report on the investigation was published in 1999. The following information taken from the report highlights some of the gross human rights violations occurring in these institutions.

The overall ratio of cots (beds) to patients was 1:1.4 indicating that floor beds were a common occurrence in many hospitals. Even in hospitals with cot to patient ratios of 1:1, many of the cots had been sent for repair, with the result that patients had to sleep on cold damp floors.

In the male wards of the hospitals at Varanasi, Indore, Murshidabad and Ahmedabad, patients were expected to urinate and defecate into an open drain in public view. Toilets in many of the hospitals were badly clogged with faeces. There were no taps in the toilets in some hospitals. Thirteen of the hospitals (35%) had very dirty toilets.

Many hospitals had problems with running water, often reflecting a scarcity of water in the state concerned. Water storage facilities were poor in 26 of the hospitals (70.2%) and there were associated water shortages. Patients sometimes had to go out of their wards in order to obtain water. Safe drinking-water was not easily available in some hospitals. A shared bucket of water was located outside each ward. During the night, when they were locked up, the patients in many hospitals had to reach through the bars of the ward in order to scoop water into a shared mug. Some of the hospitals did not provide hot water for bathing, even during the winter. Open baths were common (i.e. there were no bathrooms/washrooms and people had to take showers outdoors). Sixteen of the 37 hospitals (43.2%) had cells. In some hospitals, many patients were confined in a single cell. In others, there was one patient to a cell. Many single cells lacked water, linen, beds or toilets. Patients were locked in all the time and had to urinate and defecate in their cells.

Source: *Quality assurance in mental health*. New Delhi: National Human Rights Commission of India; 1999.

Some developing countries have taken steps to make mental health services more widely available by integrating them into primary care. Some other countries have also made mental health services available in general hospitals. Unfortunately, both ways of providing these services are only available to small proportions of the populations concerned, usually in urban centres or selected rural areas. There has been little concerted effort to use primary care as the principal vehicle for the delivery of mental health services. Box 6 and Box 7 contain examples of integrated services. Box 8 contains examples of geographical disparities in the provision of mental health services.

Primary care services are still not being used as the principal vehicle for service delivery in most countries.

Box 6. Examples from various countries of mental health services in primary care

Argentina: In Neuquen Province, cooperation between primary care general practitioners forming part of the general health sector and consulting psychologists from the mental health sector was hampered by different training paradigms. The general practitioners desired more training in mental health issues and better coordination with consulting psychiatrists and psychologists. The provincial health department responded by creating a commission on mental health which, among other things, focused on constructing a sound referral and consultation network and training primary care general practitioners and nurses in remote rural regions. In order to design an appropriate training programme the commission convened a conference for general practitioners to which professionals with diverse international experience and training in mental health issues were invited. There were representatives of nursing, psychiatry, primary care medicine, the clergy, social work, and law. The training team included people from Argentina, Chile, Guatemala, the United Kingdom, Uruguay, and the USA. After the training experience the mental health commission, which included representatives of the fields of mental health and primary care, coordinated further training and long-term follow-up of both the general practitioners and local psychologists in the primary care setting (Collins et al., 1999a). This approach to integrating mental health care into primary care operates on various levels. At the level of the provincial government there is cooperation between the mental health and primary care sectors on the mental health commission. At the primary care level there is wider intersectoral cooperation between different professions with a stake in the issues. The training programme promotes cooperation between general practitioners, nurses and social workers in the context of providing support to families, and a similar training programme has been designed for nurses (Collins et al.,1999a). In the context of the consultative approach pursued at the primary care level, some general practitioners in rural regions meet every month with traditional healers to coordinate the treatment of certain illnesses, enhance the degree to which communities trust general practitioners, and prevent dangerous dual treatments involving the use of herbs and medications (Collins et al., 1999b).

China: General primary health care services are provided by outpatient clinics in street, neighbourhood or district general hospitals (Pearson, 1992; Yan et al., 1995). There are various community services at the primary care level. They include home beds with visits from personnel attached to district or neighbourhood hospitals and nursing or supervisory care groups organized at the street level and the residents' association level (Pearson, 1992). In Shanghai there are hot-line services for adolescents and the elderly (Ji, 1995).

Botswana: Psychiatric nurses based in secondary-level district hospitals oversee a number of primary care clinics in each district. They visit these clinics regularly and meet primary care workers who have identified vulnerable cases in the community (Ben-Tovim, 1987).

Guinea-Bissau: A well-functioning primary care system with an infrastructure and paid workers was in place before the recent war. Nurses in the primary care health centres were trained to identify and treat cases of major mental disorder presenting in clinics (De Jong, 1996).

India: The Bellary district project involved the training of all categories of primary health and welfare personnel, the provision of essential psychotropic drugs, a simple record-keeping system, and a mechanism for monitoring the work of primary care personnel providing mental health care services (Murthy, 1998). Primary care centres generally provide preventive and curative services for 30 000 people and have one or two doctors and 15 to 20 basic health workers. The doctors in the clinics supervise the health workers, who visit families at home and carry out a wide array of health activities. Patients are seen in the centres without appointment. On average a consultation lasts between three and five minutes. Despite all the inputs of mental health training there still appears to be a relatively low recognition of emotional disorder by primary care doctors. This is attributable to patients presenting with somatic complaints and to the brevity of the consultations (Channabasavanna et al., 1995).

Islamic Republic of Iran: Efforts to integrate mental health care started in the late 1980s and the programme has since been extended throughout the country. There are now services for about 20 million people (Mohit et al., 1999).

Pakistan: A model of mental health care delivery integrated into primary care was initially developed in two subdistricts of Rawalpindi (Mubbashar, 1999). It is now being replicated in parts of all provinces. The component of training in mental health has been integrated into the training programme of district health development centres. These centres have been set up to build the capacity of primary care personnel so that they can handle the emerging common health problems. Under this scheme more than 2000 primary care physicians and more than 40 000 primary care personnel (including female health workers and multipurpose health workers) have received training throughout the country in a decentralized manner. More than 65 junior psychiatrists have been trained in community mental health so that they can act as resource persons in the development of community mental health programmes in their areas and provide the training, referral and evaluation support necessary for integrating mental health care into primary care. A national essential drug list has been formulated which includes all the essential neuropsychiatric drugs. Another crucial development has been the inclusion of priority mental disorders in the national health management information system. The Government has agreed to fund the integration of mental health into primary care on a national scale and a separate budget has been allocated for this purpose.

Tanzania: Rural dispensaries are provided by public, private and voluntary sources. These facilities offer basic medical services in rural regions (Ahmed et al., 1996). In some rural areas, agricultural rehabilitation villages provide sheltered employment, continuous contact with local community members, and ongoing psychosocial support from traditional healers, community health workers, and general practitioners. These community-based services provide an alternative to hospital inpatient services for long-term and medium-term patients (Kilonzo & Simmons, 1998).

Box 7. Examples from various countries of mental health services in general hospitals

Ethiopia: The services at the tertiary level have collaboratively developed a programme of mental health care at the secondary level by training psychiatric nurses. Twenty-seven regional hospitals and one health centre have opened psychiatric units, each operated by two psychiatric nurses (Alem et al., 1999).

Nepal: Secondary-level psychiatric units are located in district hospitals. The facilities at the secondary level include smaller psychiatric wards in the military hospital and two regional hospitals, and a small community mental health programme at three other regional hospitals. The mental health care units outside the capital do not include services for long-stay inpatients (Tausig & Subedi, 1997).

Tanzania: Community mental health care teams have been established in secondary-level clinics in the capital city but there are no such teams in rural areas. In both rural and urban areas, secondary-level facilities are located in psychiatric units in district general hospitals (Kilonzo & Simmons, 1998).

Tunisia: Since 1956, 300 new psychiatric beds have been provided in small psychiatric units in five general hospitals throughout the country, and the bed capacity of the only mental hospital has been halved.

Box 8. Examples from various developing countries showing the concentration of mental health services in urban areas

Botswana: Specialized mental health services are found in the capital city and regional centres, while the rural regions rely for mental health services on primary care clinics, the visits of psychiatric nurses to these clinics, and traditional healers (Ben-Tovim, 1987; Sidandi et al., 1999).

Cambodia: Although 85% of the country's population lives in rural areas there are few mental health resources other than traditional healers in these areas. There are relatively few district mental health clinics in outlying regions. Patients often travel over 300 kilometres from neighbouring districts and provinces in order to reach a clinic.

Costa Rica: Most mental health care workers are concentrated in urban settings. The rural regions are understaffed (Gallegos & Montero, 1999).

Ethiopia: All tertiary psychiatric institutions are based in the capital city, as are most psychiatrists. The regional hospitals with psychiatric units are in both urban and rural regions. There are plans to extend the psychiatric service to more district hospitals and health centres in the rural regions. There are no mental health services in primary care clinics in either urban or rural settings. Traditional healers meet the mental health needs of rural communities. It is common practice for people in rural regions to care for family members with mental disorders at home (Alem et al., 1999; Awas et al., 1999).

Former Eastern Bloc countries: Mental health services are still organized by central planning bureaucracies and there is a clear demarcation between local and central administration. Authority resides at the centre, i.e. the urban centres. Remote rural areas are forced to supply services conceived and financed by the central bureaucracy (Tomov, 1999).

Nigeria: Urban hospitals have more medical personnel and their support facilities function more efficiently than government hospitals in rural areas (Gureje et al., 1995).

Pakistan: There are residential and day care facilities for people with learning difficulties which provide social, vocational and educational activities in the big cities. However, these services are not accessible to the vast majority of rural people (Yousaf, 1997).

South Africa: There are almost 500 registered psychiatrists, but because of factors such as emigration and preferences for working in urban areas and the private sector there are areas of the country, indeed whole provinces, where there is only one psychiatrist for over 5 million people in the public sector.

Tanzania: In the rural areas the ratio of Western-trained doctors to the population is 1:20 000 while that of traditional healers to the population is 1:25. In these areas, primary mental health care still relies on medical officers, mental health nurses and auxiliaries. Psychiatrists are found only in the major urban centres with regional psychiatric facilities. The imbalance in the numbers of mental health professionals between urban and rural areas is also reflected in the presence of community mental health care teams in the capital city and their absence from rural areas.

In some countries there are good examples of intersectoral collaboration between nongovernmental organizations, academic institutions, public sector health services, informal mental health services and users, leading to the development of much-needed community-based services. At present such activities are limited to small populations in urban areas; the vast majority of rural populations have no access to such services. There is an urgent need to encourage such activities as they can provide mental health services in a manner that is acceptable to local communities. Box 9 contains examples of such intersectoral collaboration.

Nongovernmental organizations can play an important role in service provision.

Box 9. Examples of intersectoral collaboration from various countries

Cambodia: There is intersectoral cooperation between external donors and mental health services at the tertiary level. The Canadian Marcel Roy Foundation for the Children of Cambodia funded a children's mental health clinic at the tertiary mental hospital, while the International Organization for Migration supported by the Norwegian Council for Mental Health initiated a project for training doctors as psychiatrists.

Czech Republic: The FOKUS association for mental health care involves intersectoral cooperation. This service provider has become a nongovernmental organization, which allows it to receive government funds and private donations. FOKUS obtains funds from the Ministries of Social Affairs, Health, and Culture, the Labour Office, and the Prague Municipal Government, as well as from foreign and local private donor organizations. (Holmes & Koznar, 1998).

Ethiopia: Intersectoral cooperation takes place at the national level between the Ministry of Health, the University Department of Psychiatry and WHO. These bodies began a training programme for psychiatric nurses in 1986 (Alem et al., 1999).

Israel: Regional mental health boards headed by psychiatrists are responsible for supervising, coordinating and developing all mental health services and the collection of all information on mental health in each region. Each board works with a regional coordination committee that includes representatives of central government, insurers, voluntary agencies, providers and service users (Tyano & Mozes, 1998).

Romania: The Ministry of Health and Ministry of Education launched a programme in 2001 to promote health education in schools, in which mental health issues are well represented.

Tanzania: Psychiatric agricultural rehabilitation villages encapsulate an intersectoral response by local communities, the mental health sector and the traditional healing sector to the treatment and rehabilitation of people with severe mental disorders in rural areas. Patients and relatives live with a village population of farmers, fishermen and craftsmen and are treated by both the medical and traditional healing sectors. There are plans for a more formal collaboration between the traditional healing and mental health sectors, as the former could play an increased role in managing stress-related disorders in the community. Traditional healers have participated in community mental health training programmes and have shared their knowledge and skills in the management of patients with mental disorders. Plans to increase communication between the traditional healing and mental health sectors involve holding regular meetings and seminars (Kilonzo & Simmons, 1998).

Zimbabwe: The Harare City Health Department and the University of Zimbabwe Medical School are collaborating in a research project, in connection with which members of the community and primary care nurses are looking for ways of treating depressed women. Local terminology for depression and ideas on treatment were established by interviewing traditional healers and key community figures including schoolteachers, police officers, church officials and organizers of women's cooperatives. Health workers then presented the results of a survey of depressed women to community members and coined a local phrase to describe the typical pattern of symptoms of depression. The participants, who included community members, health workers and policy-makers, were divided into working groups and asked to develop recommendations for treating depressed women. They recommended that: 1) there should be a private room in primary care clinics for counselling on emotional problems; 2) a directory should be created to improve communication between helping agencies; 3) traditional healers, church leaders, teachers and the media should be used to provide education for living; 4) the detection and treatment of depression in primary care clinics should be improved (Abas et al., 1995). The programme of identification and treatment at the primary care level was integrated with a pre-existing highly developed initiative, viz. a maternal and child health programme that involved cooperation between the mental health sector and the general health sector. A more general mental health package was also integrated into the primary care system in Harare on the basis of a similar cooperative approach. Consultations between key health providers, policy-makers, academics and nongovernmental organizations occurred at the city level and a multidisciplinary research team was formed. The objective was to identify the mental disorders that occurred most frequently among persons attending for primary care, in order to develop guidelines for understanding and treating them at this level. The project involved collaboration between psychiatrists, social scientists, primary care workers, traditional and faith healers and general practitioners (Abas et al., 1995; Patel, 2000).

Developed countries rely less on mental hospitals to provide mental health care. The process of deinstitutionalization in the last three decades has led to a reduction in the numbers of patients in mental hospitals and the closure of many of these institutions. However, a different set of problems remains in these countries. The deinstitutionalization process has not been accompanied by a sufficient provision of community-based residential and occupational facilities (Thornicroft & Tansella, 1999). National constitutional structures and funding pathways of health systems have impacted on both the rate of deinstitutionalization and the provision of alternative community mental health services in various developed countries (Goodwin, 1997). Deinstitutionalization in North American and Western European countries leads to a gradual provision of community mental health services. However, these services are often inadequate and unevenly distributed nationally.

Even in developed countries, de-institutionalization has not been accompanied by an adequate provision of services in the community.

Even in developed countries there is insufficient emphasis on developing mental health services in primary care. For example, depression is a common problem in primary care settings but is still not identified or is undertreated by primary care practitioners in many such countries. There is also an emphasis on developing more specialist services, e.g. forensic services, to the detriment of general hospital-based psychiatric services. For example, in the United Kingdom there has seen a vast expansion of medium-security beds in the last few years while there is a shortage of acute general psychiatric beds and the occupancy rate is nearly 100% in many of these general psychiatric units. See Box 10 for a summary of some of the advantages and disadvantages of deinstitutionalization.

There is significant potential for using primary care services, even in developed countries.

Box 10. Advantages and disadvantages of deinstitutionalization in developed countries

Advantages

- Deinstitutionalization involves a shift in emphasis from custodial accommodation to rehabilitation programmes in community settings. It is more humane in that it avoids the detrimental psychological effects of long-term hospitalization and focuses on patients becoming reintegrated into community settings.
- It involves the prevention of new admissions by providing alternative community services and programmes that are supposedly cheaper to run. It thereby promotes efficiency and cost-effectiveness.
- It involves the release into the community of all institutional patients who have received adequate preparation. This avoids the detrimental effects of long stays such as apathy and loss of interest, and also cuts the cost of supporting patients in hospital settings for long periods of time (Thornicroft & Tansella, 1999).

Disadvantages

- Deinstitutionalization has often not resulted in the securing of adequate long-term funding for the maintenance of public mental health services in community settings (Talbott, 1978; Goodwin, 1997).
- While leading to an overall decrease in the long-stay inpatient population, deinstitutionalization has resulted in increasing numbers of readmissions, i.e. multiple short-term stays for specific patients requiring inpatient treatment (Talbott, 1978; Breakey, 1996a).
- In some instances it has led to an increase in homelessness among persons with mental disorders and to a high rate of mental disorder in prison populations.

Two main conclusions can be drawn from the experiences that have been gained.

- Firstly, mental health services pose a challenge for both developing and developed countries. However, the nature of the challenges differs. In many developing countries there is gross underprovision of resources, personnel and services. This state of affairs requires immediate attention. In developed countries some of the problems are: insufficient community reprovision; the need to promote the detection and treatment of mental disorders in primary care settings; the competing needs and demands of general psychiatric services and specialist services.

The nature of the proble differs between develope and developing countrie.

- Secondly, more expensive specialist services cannot provide a solution to these problems. Even within the resource constraints that health services confront in nearly all countries, significant improvements in the delivery of mental health services can be achieved by redirecting resources towards services that are less expensive, have reasonably good outcomes, and benefit larger proportions of populations. In practice this means emphasizing the delivery of mental health services through primary care.

An increase in specialist services will not necess improve access to ment health care.

Key points: Current status of service organization

- Very few countries have an optimal mix of services.
- In many countries there have been few concerted efforts to use primary care as the principal vehicle for the delivery of mental health services.
- Innovative service provision involving collaborative efforts of many sectors exists in many countries but is usually limited to small populations in urban areas or selected rural areas.
- In developed countries the process of deinstitutionalization has not always been accompanied by a sufficient provision of alternative community-based services.
- Mental health services pose challenges both for developing and developed countries but the nature of these challenges differs.
- More expensive and/or specialist services are not necessarily the answer to increasing access to and availability of mental health services.

4. Guidance for organizing services

No single model of service organization can meet the needs of all countries. The recommendations outlined in this section are broad principles that are likely to be applicable in most countries. Each country should adapt them to its own circumstances.

People with mental disorders often have a complex range of needs that cannot be fulfilled by the health services alone. Furthermore, different stakeholders in this field are likely to have particular perspectives that can usefully inform the development of services. People with mental disorders, their families and communities are equal partners with mental health services, and it is important that all of these stakeholders should actively communicate and collaborate with each other so as to meet the needs under consideration. Health care settings and levels of care should be organized in a way that fulfils this goal (World Health Organization, 2001).

People with mental disorders have complex needs which frequently cut across the traditional professional sectors.

4.1 Principles for the organization of services

The recommendations given below should be seen as a part of a comprehensive reorganization of services. None of the individual recommendations can succeed on its own in improving the care of people with mental disorders. The emphasis is on an integrated system of service delivery which attempts to comprehensively address the various needs of people with mental disorders. In such a system each of the distinct channels of service delivery, e.g. services in primary care and services based in general hospitals, has an important and complementary role with respect to the others. It is necessary to provide a range and variety of services that can meet needs that arise at different times.

Special attention should be given to the development of comprehensive and integrated systems of service delivery.

Failure is likely, for example, if a strategy is adopted whereby primary care staff are encouraged to perform interventions without making adequate provision for secondary care services or community services in the field of mental health. None of the strategies for service reorganization discussed below can stand on its own. Each strategy needs support and in turn will support other parts of an integrated service delivery system.

The key principles for organizing services are discussed below.

I) Accessibility: Essential mental health care should be available locally so that people do not have to travel long distances. This includes outpatient and inpatient care and other services such as rehabilitative care. An absence of services locally acts as a significant barrier to obtaining mental health care, especially for people living in remote rural areas. Services located close to persons with mental disorders can provide continuity of care in a comparatively satisfactory manner. It is difficult to address many social and psychological issues when people have to travel long distances in order to contact mental health services.

Systems of service delivery can be arranged around key principles.

II) Comprehensiveness: Mental health services should include all facilities and programmes that are required to meet the essential care needs of the populations in question. The exact mix of services required varies from place to place. It depends on social, economic and cultural factors, the characteristics of disorders and the way in which health services are organized and funded (see Section 6.2).

III) Coordination and continuity of care: Especially for people with severe mental disorders it is extremely important that services work in a coordinated manner and attempt to meet the range of social, psychological and medical care needs. This requires input from services that are not directly related to health, e.g. social services and housing services. Persons with mental disorders often find it extremely difficult to gain access to various essential services, with the result that poor outcomes occur. Mental health services should therefore perform a coordination function and prevent the fragmentation of care (see Section 7.2).

One way of addressing the need for continuity of care is to apply the sectoral or catchment area method of organizing services. During the 1960s and 1970s, health departments in North America and Western Europe divided their countries into health districts or catchment areas, i.e. they defined geographical areas with populations of between 50 000 and 250 000 (Breakey, 1996b; Thornicroft & Tansella, 1999). Catchment area health care teams covered all levels of service provision, i.e. primary, secondary and tertiary care, and were responsible for the provision of health care services for all the inhabitants of the areas concerned. Apart from the planning, budgeting and management advantages of this approach, one of the key clinical advantages is that there is an enhanced likelihood of providing continuity of care. This is of enormous benefit as many mental disorders tend to be long-lasting and require ongoing care for substantial periods.

IV) Effectiveness: Service development should be guided by evidence of the effectiveness of particular interventions. For example, there is a growing evidence base of effective interventions for many mental disorders, among them depression, schizophrenia and alcohol dependence. This evidence is reviewed in Section 7.1. (See also World Health Organization, 2001a.)

V) Equity: People's access to services of good quality should be based on need. In order to ensure equity it is necessary to address issues of access and geographical disparities. Equity should be taken into consideration when priorities are being set. All too often the people most in need of services are the least likely or the least able to demand services and are thus likely to be ignored when priorities are being set.

VI) Respect for human rights: Services should respect the autonomy of persons with mental disorders, should empower and encourage such persons to make decisions affecting their lives and should use the least restrictive types of treatment.

4.2 Establishment of an optimal mix of services

Nearly all the service delivery models discussed in Section 4 have both strengths and weaknesses. The key issue for service planners is to determine the optimal mix of services and the level of provision of particular service delivery channels. The absolute need for various services differs greatly between countries but the relative needs for different services, i.e. the proportions of different services as parts of total mental health service provision, are broadly the same in many countries. Services should be planned in a holistic fashion so as to create an optimal mix.

Planners should provide a range of services.

Services should be planned in a holistic fashion so as to create an optimal mix.

Figure 2 shows the relationships between the different service components. It is clear that the most numerous services ought to be self-care management, informal community mental health services and community-based mental health services provided by primary care staff, followed by psychiatric services based in general hospitals and formal community mental health services, and lastly by specialist mental health services. The emphasis placed on delivering mental health treatment and care through services based in general hospitals or community mental health services should be determined by the strengths of the current mental health or general health system, as well as by cultural and socioeconomic variables.

There is little justification for including the kind of services provided by mental hospitals when consideration is being given to the optimal mix of services. Mental hospitals essentially provide long-stay custodial care. With the development of a range of community-based services and specialist services there is no need for mental hospitals. There will always be a need for long-stay facilities for an extremely small proportion of patients, even if there is good provision of community-based services. However, most of these patients can be accommodated in small units in the community, with an approximation to community living as far as is possible. Alternatively, small long-stay wards in hospitals can also provide other specialist services. (See also Planning and Budgeting to Deliver Services for Mental Health.) Large-scale custodial institutional care as provided by mental hospitals is not justified either by its costs, its effectiveness or the quality of care provided.

With the development of a range of community-based and specialist services there is no need for mental hospitals.

Figure 2: Optimal mix of different mental health services

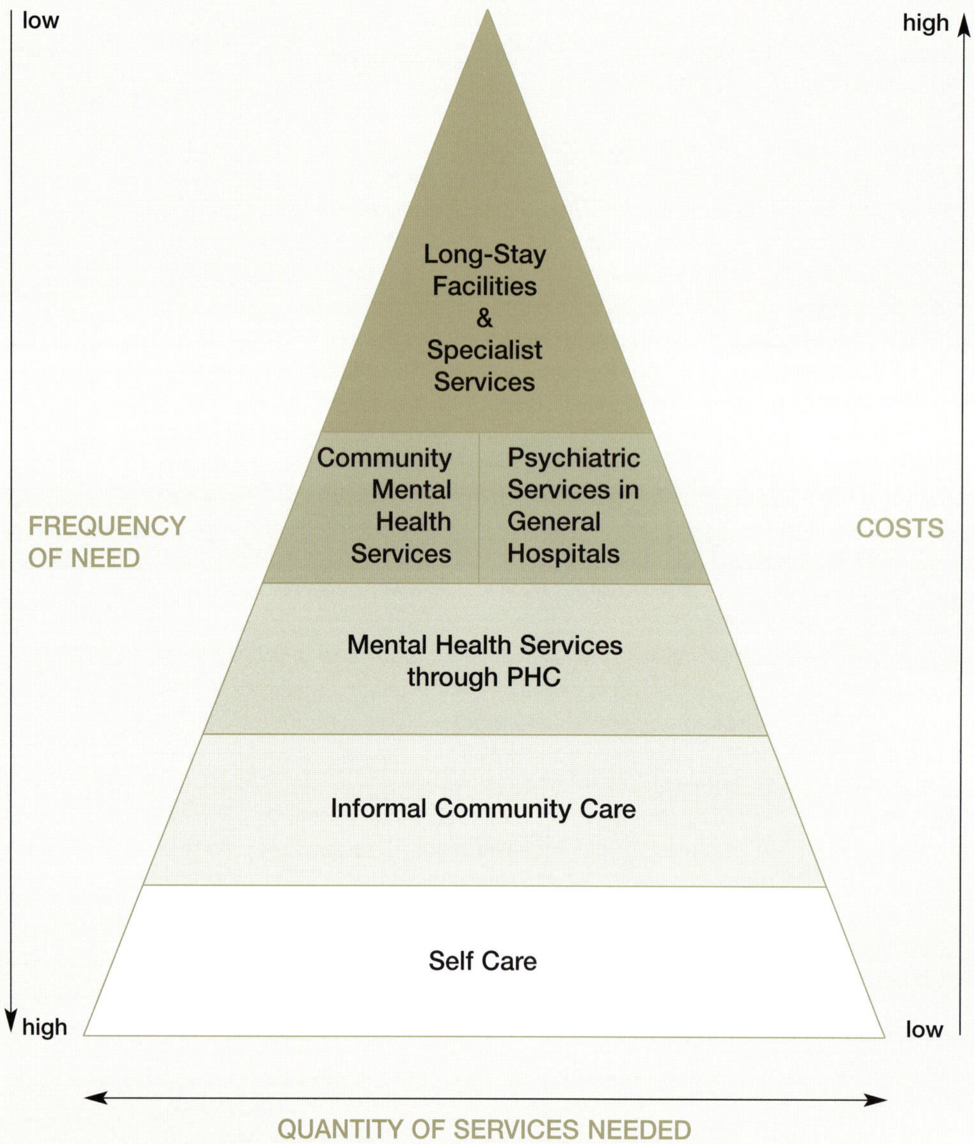

4.3 Integration of mental health services into general health services

In order to overcome the difficulties associated with segregated services it is necessary to integrate mental health services into general health services. Integrated care helps to reduce the stigma associated with seeking help from stand-alone mental health services. In developing countries with acute shortages of mental health professionals the delivery of mental health services through general health care is the most viable strategy for increasing access to mental health care among underserved populations. Furthermore, mental disorders and physical health problems are very closely associated and often influence each other. For example, people with common mental disorders such as depression and anxiety frequently present with somatic symptoms to general health care services. An integrated service encourages the early identification and treatment of such disorders and thus reduces disability. Other potential benefits include possibilities for providing care in the community and opportunities for community involvement in care.

Integrated care helps to reduce stigma, addresses shortages of human resources and improves access to mental health services for underserved populations.

Integration can be pursued at all levels. At the clinical level, mental health care can be integrated into the primary, secondary and tertiary levels of general health care. This may be accompanied by managerial and administrative integration as well as the development of integrated information systems. (See also *Planning and Budgeting to Deliver Services for Mental Health*.) For example, mental health professionals working in the general health care system may have a management structure (line management) that is quite separate from that of the general health staff. This occasionally creates difficulties in their day-to-day working and in their relationships with colleagues in the general health system. Managerial integration can help to resolve some of these issues.

Information systems for general health are separate from mental health information systems in many countries. This creates difficulties for planners and managers in the general health system because they plan services without appreciating the burden of mental disorders. The integration of mental health information systems with general health information systems can improve the total health situation in a country. It can also help advocate for better mental health services by making the substantial burden of mental disorders obvious to health planners. However, some information specific to mental health should be available in order to enable the appropriate planning and evaluation of mental health services. This may require the modification of general health information systems so as to include the recording of mental health service provision and attendance by people with mental disorders.

Full integration, involving clinical, administrative, managerial and information systems, has certain drawbacks. Mental health services may prefer to retain a degree of separation, e.g. separate management structures at lower management levels. A degree of separation may help to protect budgets for mental health care and to preserve the professional identity of mental health staff.

Full integration has its advantages and drawbacks

When choosing between full and partial integration, countries should assess the potential benefits and disadvantages of each and should take account of the way in which primary care services are organized. In most situations, strategic planning for service integration is necessary (Box 11).

Box 11. Strategic planning for the integration of mental health services

Major issues in strategic planning include the following:

(I) Working out how the mainstreaming of mental health into the general health delivery system is to be carried out. This involves setting out organizational changes and delineating responsibilities.

(II) Budgeting for new posts, physical facilities, equipment and transport.

(III) Planning for mental health teams and their responsibilities.

(IV) Preparing job descriptions for various professionals and supporting staff at each level of care, e.g. primary care workers, mental health care workers, and supervisors, and specifying their responsibilities in connection with the coverage of the various mental health conditions that are being targeted.

(V) Planning for: the institutional training of personnel requiring skills; on-the-job training; continuing medical education; the insertion of mental health material into the curricula of health and health-related training institutions.

(VI) Strategies for mobilizing and involving community members and consumers at every level of activity.

At a basic level, integration into general health care involves:

- the integration of mental health services into primary care settings;
- the integration of mental health services into general hospitals;
- the development of links between primary care and secondary services based in general hospitals;
- the integration of mental health care into other established health and social programmes.

4.3.1 Integration of mental health services into primary care settings

In countries with limited resources the integration of mental health care into the general health delivery system necessarily involves integration into primary care. First and foremost this requires the training of primary care staff. Primary care workers have to assume increasing responsibilities for the promotion of mental health and the provision of mental health services. Health workers in training institutions and those already in the field have to be oriented towards the provision of services in the primary care setting. They also have to be equipped with knowledge and skills enabling them to provide such services. Primary care workers may resist taking on these roles. For example, they may question their role in managing mental disorders. They may be uncomfortable about dealing with mental disorders or they may ignore and withdraw from working with people who have such disorders. Clinical outcomes, which are highly dependent on the knowledge and skills of primary care staff, would consequently be unsatisfactory. Furthermore, the acceptability of the service would be reduced if poorly trained staff ignored mental disorders or did not pay equal attention to mental and physical disorders. Solutions to these problems are considered in Section 9.

Primary care staff need training and skills in order to be able to treat mental disorders.

Primary care workers should be prepared to take part in this process. Their tasks, obligations and responsibilities should be outlined as they participate actively in them. They should be trained in the promotion of mental health and in the prevention and management of priority mental disorders. The training should include all categories of health workers and other workers whose work touches on the mental health of the community, e.g. security officers and receptionists in health facilities.

The training materials should include appropriate selections from those suggested for the planning team at the national level as well as other materials available locally or developed for the programme in question in order to meet the specific needs of the community. A guide on such training is available (World Health Organization, 1982).

The time factor has to be considered if primary care staff are to devote themselves adequately to mental health work. Primary care staff are overburdened in many countries, being expected to deliver multiple health care programmes that are mainly concerned with physical disorders. In such situations it is necessary to increase the numbers of primary care staff so that they can take on additional mental health work. (See *Planning and Budgeting to Deliver Services for Mental Health*.)

More primary care staff are needed in many countries if integration is to succeed.

Primary care staff have to be adequately supervised if integration is to succeed. Mental health professionals should be regularly available to primary care staff to give advice on the management and treatment of people with mental disorders. Regular supervision cannot be replaced by a system of referral to secondary and tertiary care. The absence of supervision can lead to a high rate of such referral for even minor problems that could be dealt with by primary care staff if they were supervised on site. A member of the mental health team in the secondary care services could visit the primary care team on a weekly or fortnightly basis to provide supervision. The mental health professional should be available to discuss difficulties in management and to provide advice on interventions to be carried out by primary care staff. This model of supervision has worked well in India (Murthy, 1998).

Other issues that need to be addressed include the provision of an adequate infrastructure, the availability of equipment and, most importantly, the availability of psychotropic medication. The delineation of a few targeted mental disorders to be treated at the primary care level simplifies the requirements for types of medicines. A list of medicines can be drawn up in accordance with WHO recommendations on essential drugs at various levels of care. All major categories can be made available at all levels, with a narrower range of choices at the primary care level. Bulk purchasing of generic medicines

The infrastructure and human resources must be adequate if integration into general health care is to succeed.

ensures low costs and continuous supplies throughout the year. This approach also simplifies training, as primary care workers only need to be proficient and skilled in the use of a few selected drugs. (See *Planning and Budgeting to Deliver Services for Mental Health* and *Mental Health Financing*.)

4.3.2 Integration of mental health services into general hospitals

Mental health services based in general hospitals can provide secondary-level care to patients in the community and services to those who are admitted for physical disorders and require mental health interventions. Integration into general hospitals requires facilities and human resources. (See *Planning and Budgeting to Deliver Services for Mental Health*.) The required facilities include beds for the management of acute mental disorders, outpatient facilities, equipment for specialized tests, e.g. psychological tests, equipment for specialized treatments, and medication.

The required human resources include specialist mental health staff such as psychiatrists, psychologists, psychiatric nurses and social workers. These staff have to take responsibility for the training and supervision of primary care workers. Some of these specialist staff may not be sufficiently oriented towards primary mental health care and community-based service delivery and will themselves require training.

4.3.3 Establishment of links between primary, secondary and tertiary care

Links between primary care and other levels of health care are essential

Primary health care is both an entry point and a referral point for mental health care and prevention. In order to address the needs of persons with mental disorders for health care and social support a clear referral and linkage system should be in place. It should be operated in consultation with the district and regional levels. Regular meetings of service providers should be held in order to review and improve the referral system and to evaluate how the needs of patients are being met.

Even where specialist mental health services are well developed it is important to improve coordination between them and primary care. If this is not done, care is often duplicated or poorly coordinated and delays occur when primary care workers seek help with patients in crisis.

4.3.4 Integration of mental health care into other established health and social programmes

Integration with other he and social programmes may help to overcome resource difficulties.

In developing countries, other basic health priorities compete with mental health for funding. (See *Mental Health Policy, Plans and Programmes*.) Instead of competing, mental health programmes should collaborate with other health programmes. For example, programmes aimed at tackling maternal depression can usefully become part of a wider reproductive health programme. HIV/AIDS programmes offer another opportunity to increase the coverage of mental health services to vulnerable populations. Such collaborative approaches should also be extended to programmes that are not directly related to health, e.g. women's mental health issues could be covered in programmes tackling domestic violence.

4.4 Creation of formal and informal community mental health services

Formal community men health services are the community counterpart of secondary care servic based in general hospita

Formal community mental health services are the community counterpart of secondary care services based in general hospitals. These include, for example, day centres for persons with severe mental illness who have been discharged from hospitals, hospital diversion programmes, crisis teams, group homes, halfway houses and case management services. More examples of formal community services are given in Box 12. For many developing countries it will not be immediately possible to develop all these services. In such circumstances, planners should decide which services are immediate priorities and should concentrate efforts and resources on developing them. Other services may be developed in a phased manner over time.

In many developing countries, moreover, some of these community-based services, e.g. halfway homes or group homes, may not be needed to the extent that they are required in developed countries because of the availability of good family support. This is not to suggest that families should bear the entire burden of caring for persons with severe mental disorders. However, community services should be designed to support families in their attempts to care for relatives with mental disorders.

Families are an important resource and they need active support from community services.

Developing countries should also use existing networks of nongovernmental organizations in order to provide some community-based services. These may include clubhouses, support groups, employment or rehabilitation workshops, sheltered workshops, supervised work placements, and staffed and unstaffed residential accommodation. Examples from Tanzania and Zimbabwe (Box 9) illustrate the use of available resources to provide community-based services. Boxes 12 and 13 provide other examples of the use of formal resources, e.g. nongovernmental organizations, and informal resources, e.g. neighbours and religious leaders, for providing community-based services.

Nongovernmental organizations are another useful resource.

Box 12. Innovative formal and informal community mental health services

China: Psychiatric care units consist of patients' neighbours, retired workers, and family members who assist with the care of mental patients (Pearson, 1992).

China, India, and Malaysia: Governments contract with nongovernmental organizations to provide care for childless elderly people in small residential homes (Levkoff et al., 1995).

India: Teachers are trained as counsellors in order to provide therapeutic interventions for children in schools (Nikapota, 1991). Lay volunteers provide crisis intervention services in some of the major Indian cities (Murthy, 2000).

Mongolia: Community-based day centres in traditional Mongolian tented and portable round houses called gers were started in 2000 on the grounds of district health centres in the Songinokhairkhan and Chingletei Districts of Ulan Bator. The most significant achievement in Chingletei was the setting up of a canteen in the day centre for use by medical and dental staff. The staff constructed benches and tables from broken furniture and used old crockery and cutlery from the hospital or from their own homes in setting up the canteen. Notwithstanding the significant stigma and exclusion faced by persons with mental disorders in Mongolia, medical and nursing staff of this health centre willingly ate in the canteen (World Health Organization, 2000).

Box 13. Meeting mental health needs in underresourced settings: innovations of nongovernmental organizations in India

Nongovernmental organizations have gained considerable experience in health care in India, notably in reproductive and child health services and research. In recent years a growing number of nongovernmental organizations have begun to develop innovative programmes for mental health care. In 1999 an attempt to coordinate nongovernmental organizations working in mental health programmes identified more than 50 initiatives across the country. The most common ones involved rehabilitation, the empowerment of persons with severe mental disorders, and the provision of schools for children with mental retardation. However, the range of nongovernmental organizations has grown considerably in keeping with a growing awareness of the breadth of problems associated with mental disorders, e.g. substance abuse, mental disorders in children, dementia and violence. The four nongovernmental organizations profiled below work in different areas of mental health, integrate research, training and service delivery, and collaborate actively with other sectors of the health and social welfare systems. All have relied on funding from a range of sources including individual and corporate donors, foundations, donor agencies and the Government.

The **Schizophrenia Research Foundation**, located in the southern city of Chennai, is one of India's best-known providers of comprehensive integrated services for persons affected by severe mental disorders. It was founded in 1984 by medical professionals working in a local medical school. It now provides community, outpatient, day care and residential care services for patients with severe mental disorders, including a range of psychosocial rehabilitation services. It plays a leading role in advocacy for the rights of persons with mental disorders, particularly for the formal acknowledgement of the disability produced by mental illness. It is one of the country's leading agencies conducting research into all aspects of schizophrenia. Its Madras Longitudinal Study is the most widely cited study of its kind on the outcome of schizophrenia in a developing country. The Foundation is a WHO Collaborating Centre for Research and Training in Mental Health.

The Sangath Society is located in the state of Goa on the west coast of India. It was founded in 1996 by a team of health professionals working in the field of child and adolescent development. In five years it has become the leading provider of community-based multidisciplinary child and family guidance services in the region, with more than 350 referrals a year. The Society has extended services from the clinic to the community with programmes aimed at improving child development outcomes, e.g. early intervention for high-risk babies, and to schools with programmes for improving awareness and teaching methods for children with different abilities. It actively collaborates with government departments, academic institutions and other nongovernmental organizations with a view to maximizing the potential for development of every child. It is a leading agency for research on women's mental health and adolescent health, and has also been the coordinating agency for the country's largest randomized control trial on the treatment of depression in general health care.

The **T.T. Ranganathan Clinical Research Foundation** was founded in 1980 by a woman whose husband had suffered gravely from the consequences of a severe alcohol addiction. This Foundation has pioneered a range of programmes for combating alcohol addiction, with services delivered at every level of care from the community to a fully equipped hospital. The Foundation's major innovation has consisted of outreach camps that are run for periods of two weeks to provide services for alcohol dependence in rural areas. Services are thus taken directly to communities, and individuals are not expected to travel to distant cities for specialized care. The Foundation's TTK Hospital, providing a range of medical and psychological therapies for alcohol dependence, has treated over 10 000 patients since its inception in collaboration with the United Nations Drug Control Programme. The hospital was recently recognized by WHO as a Regional Resource Training Centre.

Ashagram is a nongovernmental organization located in the Barwani District of the state of Madhya Pradesh in Western India. This is one of the poorest regions in the country, with high levels of illiteracy, severe environmental degradation and a large tribal population. Ashagram was founded in the 1980s by lay persons as a resettlement colony for people disabled by leprosy. Since then it has become a vibrant community with primary education, comprehensive health care facilities and diverse income-generating units. Mental health services were initiated in 1996 for persons with severe mental disorders. The community participatory model was used to ensure that services were accessible and in keeping with local cultural norms. The organization was largely run by mental health workers from local villages who had received a basic education. The programme on mental health was run alongside services for persons with physical disabilities. When it was necessary for a person with a mental disorder to be admitted to hospital, therefore, he or she would enter a ward used by other patients. The mental health programme has now been extended to cover common mental disorders.

Source: Patel V, Thara R, eds. *Meeting mental health needs in developing countries: NGO innovations in India*. Sage India (in press).

4.5 Limitation of dedicated mental hospitals

Mental hospitals are expensive to run and maintain. They produce poor clinical outcomes, they are associated with increased rather than decreased disability, they stigmatize patients, families and all people with mental disorders and they are associated with violations of human rights. It is therefore important to reduce dependence on mental hospitals as providers of mental health care. Deinstitutionalization is consequently a necessary part of reforming the delivery of mental health services.

De-institutionalization is not an immediate event but a planned process.

However, deinstitutionalization does not simply mean discharging people from long-stay hospitals. It is a process involving significant and systematic changes whereby the delivery of services becomes predominantly community-based rather than institutional. Community provision of services has to go hand-in-hand with reducing the numbers of people in mental hospitals. In the long run the savings from the closure of mental hospitals can be expected to compensate for increased expenditure on community-based services. In the transition period, however, services have to incur double running costs. (See *Mental Health Financing*.)

Deinstitutionalization has to address the potentially negative effects of transferring functions of the traditional mental hospital into the community. These are described in Box 14. In addition, the following activities and services should be in place before patients are transferred from hospitals to communities.

De-institutionalization should be preceded by the development of alternative community-based services.

I) Mental health services should be available in primary care facilities. This requires the training of family doctors, nurses and other primary care workers to identify and treat mental disorders.
II) Beds, facilities and specialist staff should be provided in general hospitals or in the community for the management of acute relapses requiring short-term hospitalization.
III) Staff in existing mental hospitals should be retrained to take up positions in general health care settings, including the supervision of primary care staff and the provision of mental health services in general hospitals.
IV) Psychotropic medication should be available in primary care and general hospital settings.
V) Formal and informal community mental health services should be introduced in order to help with community rehabilitation.

Once the above community-based alternatives are in place, deinstitutionalization can proceed in the following stages.

I) As a first step, all new admissions to mental hospitals should be stopped and the patients concerned should be directed to psychiatric units in general hospitals.
II) It is necessary to work with the families of patients due for discharge in order to provide both the families and the patients with help and support when discharge occurs.
III) Discharge should begin with the least disabled patients and should gradually move on to patients with increasing degrees of disability.

A minority of patients with severe mental disorders and severe disability require supervised support for 24 hours a day. These patients can also be moved into small community-based residential units with 24-hour nursing and other staff supervision if these are available.

Deinstitutionalization requires strong commitment on the part of planners, managers and clinicians. Moreover, agreement is necessary among all the stakeholders regarding the pace and timing of the process. Experience gained in Brazil shows that deinstitutionalization can succeed even if resources are limited (Box 15). Experience gained in the United Kingdom shows that community-based care for long-stay institutional patients can enhance their quality of life if there is a well-planned and well-resourced reprovision programme (Leff & Treiman, 2000). Service providers can be provided with financial incentives for meeting time-bound targets in both the development of alternative community services and the discharge of patients from long-stay institutions. Such financial incentives include increased budgetary allocations for community-based services, the provision of additional finances for the community resettlement of long-stay patients from institutions, and incentives offered to community mental health agencies for reducing bed usage. (See *Mental Health Financing* and *Planning and Budgeting to Deliver Services for Mental Health*.)

Strong commitment is required from all relevant stakeholders.

Box 14. Effects of transferring functions of the traditional mental hospital to community care

Functions of traditional mental hospitals	Effects of transfer to community care
Physical assessment and treatment	More appropriate treatment in primary care or general hospital health services
Active treatment for short-term and intermediate stays	Treatment maintained or improved but results may not be generalizable
Long-term custody	Usually improved in residential homes for those who need a high level of long-term support
Protection from exploitation	Some patients continue to be vulnerable to physical, sexual and financial exploitation
Day care and outpatient services	May be improved if locally accessible services are developed, or may deteriorate if they are not; negotiation of responsibilities is often necessary between health and social care agencies
Occupational, vocational and rehabilitation services	Improved in normal settings
Shelter, clothing, nutrition and basic income	At risk, so responsibilities and coordination should be clarified
Respite for families and carers	Usually unchanged; place of treatment at home, offset by potential for increased professional support to family
Research and training	New opportunities arise through decentralization

Source: Thornicroft G, Tansella M (2000). *Balancing community-based and hospital-based mental health care: the new agenda*. Geneva: World Health Organization.

Box 15. Examples of models of deinstitutionalization in practice

Brazil

Since 1991 there has been a 30% reduction in the number of psychiatric beds. From 1997 to 2001 there was an increase from 176 to 295 in the number of community-based mental health centres, called psychosocial care centres. Various projects have been carried out in the South-Eastern Region, which has the country's highest gross domestic product. In the State of São Paulo, the City of Santos, with a population of over 400 000, had a highly profitable private psychiatric hospital with an authorized capacity of 260 patients. In fact, it was housing 575 mental patients, many of them hospitalized for alcoholism. Numerous accusations of mistreatment and death through violence led the State Government to carry out an evaluation of the hospital in 1989, on the basis of which the hospital was closed. Five mental health centres, called psychosocial attention centres, were established, similar to the model used in Trieste, Italy. With the participation of users' associations and public functionaries this chain of centres evolved to the point where workshops were set up to provide the patients with paid work. The psychiatric hospital was eventually closed. This experience is still one of the most important in the process of change in Brazil (Alves & Valentini, 2002).

Cuba

The development of mental health services in Cuba is a good example of the organization of services with different models over the last 50 years.

- **Asylum model (until 1959):** Mental health services were scarce. There was only 1 psychiatrist per 150 000 population. The services were centralized in Havana and were mainly in large mental hospitals (1 bed per 2200 population).

- **Hospital model (1960 to 1986):** Mental health services were integrated into the national health system and resources were increased and decentralized to the whole country so as to improve access, coverage and quality. Psychiatric services in mental and general hospitals were transformed into therapeutic communities. Attention was paid to the development of human resources. The number of psychiatric beds increased. There were 11 mental hospitals, 15 psychiatric services in general hospitals and 4 psychiatric services in paediatric hospitals.

- **Ambulatory and primary care model (1987 to 1995):** Some mental health services were incorporated into primary care, 20 crisis intervention units were created and two psychiatric outpatient clinics were developed in municipalities, outside the general hospitals. Meanwhile, 30 day hospitals started to function and the number of psychiatric services increased to 23 in general hospitals and 10 in paediatric hospitals. The number of psychiatric beds increased to 1 per 1100 population. The policy of human resources development, introduced in the previous period, led to a significant increase in the number of psychiatrists (1 per 9000 population).

- **Community psychiatry model (from 1996):** The ambulatory and primary care model were seen to be in need of improvement because they failed to modify psychiatric epidemiology, they showed a poor cost-benefit ratio, consumers were dissatisfied and there was poor participation of the population. Through the participation of multiple stakeholders a new policy was formulated with the community mental health centres as the core element of the services. These centres are staffed by multidisciplinary teams (including psychiatrists) and they use any infrastructure that is available at the local level (health facilities, schools, factories, community facilities, etc.). They are well connected with primary care centres (family doctors and nurses) and with various organizations belonging to sectors other than the health sector. By the end of 1999 it had been possible to accredit 111 community mental health centres. This strategy has allowed an understanding of the needs of the population in each locality, the development of appropriate action plans and a reduction in the demand for inpatient treatment (Barrientos, 2001).

Key points: Recommendations for the organization of services

- Service planners should aim to have a range of mental health services.

- The absolute need for various services varies between countries but the relative needs for different services are similar in many countries.

- The integration of mental health services into primary care is a viable strategy for increasing access to mental health care in many countries.

- Integration into primary health care requires the training of primary care staff in the identification and treatment of mental disorders.

- In some countries, primary care staff are already overburdened and the integration of mental health care into primary care, requires an increase in the absolute numbers of primary care staff.

- The integration of mental health services into general hospitals requires specialist mental health professionals in such hospitals and the provision of infrastructural and other facilities.

- The integration of mental health services into existing general health and social care programmes targeted at vulnerable populations represents a useful strategy for overcoming resource constraints and increasing the reach of mental health services.

- It is necessary to establish community-based mental health services in countries if integration and deinstitutionalization are to succeed.

- Countries should consider using existing networks of services, especially those provided by nongovernmental organizations.

- Large mental hospitals are not justified by their costs, their effectiveness or the quality of care provided.

- Deinstitutionalization does not just involve discharging patients from long-stay hospitals. It is a process of reorienting the delivery of services mainly from a predominantly institutional perspective to a community-based perspective.

- Deinstitutionalization should follow, not precede, the establishment of community-based alternative services.

- A small proportion of patients require long-stay facilities and they can be accommodated in small units in the community or in small long-stay wards in hospitals.

5. Key issues in the organization of mental health services

The above recommendations for organizing mental health services have to take certain key issues into account. These include the evidence base for mental health interventions, the unique needs of people with mental disorders, the way communities and patients access services, and other important structural issues such as the need for intersectoral collaboration.

5.1 **Evidence-based care**

The evidence base for some commonly recommended service provision strategies is reviewed below.

There is clear evidence that, for many disorders, community-based treatm gives substantially bette outcomes than inpatient treatment..

5.1.1 **Community-based treatment and care without hospital admission**

Eleven studies in developed countries have compared the effects of community-based treatment with those of standard inpatient care (Braun et al., 1981; Conway et al., 1994). The results are given in Table 1, where + indicates significantly better outcomes than in controls and = indicates no difference between treatments and controls. Not all studies measured the same variables. The last three studies involved multidisciplinary teams, 24-hour access, crisis intervention, patient advocacy, continuing care and non-institutional residential support or day centres as components of their community programmes. Table 1 shows that community-based treatment was associated with substantially better outcomes than inpatient treatment and care.

Table 1. **Studies comparing the effects of community-based treatment with those of standard inpatient care**

Study	Global symptom-atology	Psychosocial adjustment	Admission/ readmission rates	Length of stay in hospital	Patient satisfaction	Less medication	Employment	Family burden
1	+	+						
2			+	+	+		+	+
3			+	+	+		+	+
4	+	+	+			+	+	
5	+	+	+			+	+	
6	+	+	+			+	+	
7	+	+			+			
8	+	+			+	=	+	
9	+	+	+		+			
10	+	+	+		+			
11	=	=			+			

5.1.2 **Hospital admissions followed by community based treatment**

Thirteen controlled studies in developed countries have compared the use of shorter hospital stays or substituted day care with control patients who received long-term hospital care (Braun P et al 1981). Table 2 indicates that if admitted to hospital, shorter stays are as effective as longer stays.

Table 2. **Studies comparing the outcomes of short hospital stay or substituted day care with those of long-term hospital care**

Study	Global symptomatology	Psychosocial adjustment	Admission/ readmission rates	Length of stay in hospital	Employment	Family burden
1	=	+	=	+		
2	-				+	=
3	=	+	=	+		
4				+		
5				+		
6	+	+	=		+	+
7	=	=	=			
8	= (one year)					=
9	= (two years)	=				=
10	=	–				
11	=					
12			+	+		
13						

5.1.3 Community-based treatment and care for persons with severe mental disorders

De-institutionalization is associated with good outcomes.

A selection of five valid studies comparing controls with community-based care for persons with severe mental disorders who had previously been hospitalized for extended periods is presented in Table 3 (Braun et al., 1981), where + indicates a significantly better outcome than in controls and = indicates no difference from controls. Table 3 shows that community-based treatment and care were associated with improved outcomes.

Table 3. **Studies comparing controls with community-based care for those persons with severe mental disorders who had previously been hospitalized for extended periods**

Study	Global symptomatology	Social functioning	Admission/ readmission rates	Independent living	Employment	Family burden
1	=					
2	=			+	+	
3	+			+	+	+
4		+	+			
5	+	+				

5.1.4 Treatment of major mental disorders

There is substantial evidence demonstrating that the major mental disorders can be effectively treated and that relapse rates can be reduced by a combination of psychopharmacological and psychosocial rehabilitation interventions. In the treatment of schizophrenia, for example, a combination of regular medication and family interventions can reduce the rate of relapse from nearly 50% to less than 10% (Leff & Gamble, 1995; Dixon & Lehman, 1995).

Programmes aimed at reducing depression in mothers and thus at reducing adverse outcomes for their children have proved effective. They can be delivered in primary care settings by, for example, health visitors and community health workers (Cooper & Murray, 1998). There is also evidence to show that depression can be effectively treated by primary care personnel using a combination of medications and psychotherapy or counselling (Mynors-Wallis et al., 1996; Schulberg et al., 1996; Ward et al., 2000; Bower et al., 2000; Sriram et al., 1990).

Depression can be managed effectively in primary care.

A full description of cost-effective interventions is available (World Health Organization, 2001a).

5.2 Episodic care versus continuing care

Health systems in most countries, and especially those in developing countries, are designed to provide health care on the basis of the throughput model. This emphasizes the importance of vigorous treatment of acute episodes in the expectation that most patients will make a reasonably complete recovery without a need for ongoing care until the next acute episode, if there is one. The model works well for a narrow range of communicable diseases and is defended on the grounds that it helps to ration expert resources and discourages dependency. It is, however, ill-suited to the needs of many people with mental disorders whose conditions are only partially responsive to treatment and whose medical condition is inexorably linked to difficulties in daily living.

Many mental disorders, especially those with a chronic course or with a relapsing-remitting pattern, are better managed by services that adopt a continuing care model. This emphasizes the long-term nature of the disorders and the need for a continuing therapeutic input. A continuing care approach also emphasizes the need to address the totality of patients' needs, including their social, occupational and psychological needs. Such approaches therefore require a significant degree of collaboration between different care agencies.

The continuing care moc helps to address the tota of needs of many persor with severe mental disorders.

The sectorization or catchment area method of provision is an example of organizing services so as to maintain continuity of care. The catchment area team takes responsibility for the provision of care on an ongoing basis for persons living in a designated geographical area.

Effective continuing care requires the coordination of patients' medical and social care needs in the community. In many developed countries this emphasis on coordination has led to the development of case management models of care. Case management encompasses strategies aimed at minimizing service fragmentation by establishing contact persons for the coordination of care (see Section 5.5).

5.3 Pathways to care

The pathways to care are the routes whereby people with mental disorders gain access to providers of mental health services. These pathways influence the organization of services.

In established market economies the common pathways to care include:

- the primary care system;
- referral from secondary and tertiary medical care facilities;
- referral by other sources such as schools, social workers and courts.

In developing countries the most common pathways to care include:

- village health workers;
- nurses;
- primary care clinics;
- traditional healers;
- direct access to specialist services in the public or private sector.

These pathways may hinder access to mental health services because of:

Established pathways to care and treatment may hinder access to services and lead to poor outcomes.

- low awareness of available services;
- a lack of well-organized primary mental health care;
- inadequate links between services;
- a lack of knowledge among rural populations about the causes of and treatments for mental disorders, resulting in the underutilization of mental health services;
- inadequate mental health training of general practitioners and traditional healers, contributing to low rates of detection, treatment and referral of mental disorders in traditional and primary care settings;
- a failure of mental health services to actively identify cases in the community, users being required to find and access available pathways;
- difficulty in accessing specialist services, partly associated with the need for professional referral to specialist programmes.

These barriers often lead to negative outcomes, such as delays in seeking or obtaining care until full-blown disorders have developed with a higher likelihood of poor long-term outcomes and greater costs of treatment.

Service planners should organize services so as to overcome these barriers, improve access and thus reduce the duration and severity of disability caused by mental disorders. Some countries have attempted to overcome these barriers by improving communication with local communities in order to increase the visibility of formal mental health services. Communities need information about the availability of mental health services. Such information should be disseminated through both formal and informal means. Community health workers and primary care workers can actively promote mental health issues and undertake early identification work in communities. The creation of clear referral mechanisms from primary care to secondary mental health services and vice versa is another strategy for reducing barriers to care (see Section 9).

5.4 Geographical disparities

It is necessary to address geographical disparities.

In all developing countries there is an imbalance of resources between mental health services in rural settings and those in urban settings. Innovative rural programmes are therefore necessary in countries lacking many of the basic mental health resources, e.g. primary care centres and psychiatric units. Health care personnel in many countries are reluctant to serve in remote rural areas because of a lack of general facilities. It may be necessary to consider providing financial or other professional incentives in order to induce staff to serve in remote areas. In countries with reasonable transport links an outreach service from primary or secondary mental health services to rural and remote areas may represent a feasible option for extending services. Yet another strategy involves training village-level workers in the basic identification of mental disorders and providing them with weekly or monthly supervision by visiting mental health professionals (see Section 10, Barrier 2 and solutions).

5.5 Service-led care versus needs-led care

In order to be effective, mental health services have to focus on the needs of patients with mental disorders and provide services to meet these needs. However, mental health services often encounter problems in the implementation of this well-understood and well-accepted principle of care.

Many services, including those of health care, social work, social security and housing, are arranged hierarchically with distinctions between service levels and service providers. These distinctions include separate managerial arrangements, separate budgets and differences in the modes of entry into services, e.g. referral systems. These services have often developed independently from each other. For example, health care budgets are held and implemented by health ministries while housing budgets are controlled and disbursed by housing ministries. In most cases these organizational arrangements are based primarily on a managerial perspective and users have to adjust to the peculiar structures of the services they need to access.

These organizational arrangements cause considerable difficulties for people with mental disorders. In theory, users should be able to move seamlessly, in accordance with their needs, between different service levels and service providers. But for people with mental disorders these organizational structures often become barriers to obtaining the care they need.

Service organization sometimes does not tak[e] into account the needs of people with mental disorders.

In order to address this problem it is essential that services be designed on a needs-led basis rather than on a service-led basis. This means adapting services to users' needs, and not the other way round.

The coordination of care is an important aspect of developing needs-led care. In many instances it is necessary for mental health services to link with and coordinate the activities of agencies outside the health sector, e.g. housing, employment and social security, in order to obtain the services required by patients.

The implementation of a needs-led service structure does not always require additional financial resources. It does, however, require a commitment to adapt services to patients' needs. If, for example, patients have to travel long distances to clinics, their needs can be met if the clinics are opened in the afternoon rather than in the morning. This has no financial implications for the services.

A needs-led model of service provision can effectively implemented.

The key points are that the needs of populations should be reviewed locally, consideration should be given to how services are accessed locally, and service provision should be modified so as to maximize the probability of meeting patients' needs.

The key point is that services should review t[he] needs of local populatio[n] order to maximize the probability of meeting th[e] needs of people with me[ntal] disorders.

There are moves towards needs-led models of service provision in many industrialized countries and in some developing countries. Examples include brokerage models and assertive case management for patients with severe mental disorders (Stein and Test, 1980) and a model for psychosocial rehabilitation adopted in rural settings in Tanzania (Box 9). These models are an acknowledgment that patients' needs should be considered first and foremost and that the organization of services should be adapted in order to meet them.

5.6 Collaboration within and between sectors

People with mental disorders have complex needs that cut across service sectors. It is unlikely that the health sector alone can meet all the needs of these people for social care. In developing countries, moreover, the mental health sector may be relatively small in comparison with the other sectors that may be able to supplement its activities. Collaboration is therefore essential if the outcomes of mental disorders are to be improved.

Collaboration within and between sectors is essential for meeting the complex needs of persons with mental disorders.

Collaboration is needed within the health sector, i.e. intrasectoral collaboration, and outside the health sector, i.e. intersectoral collaboration.

Collaboration within the health sector involves links with primary and secondary mental health care, links between the mental health sector and the general health sector at the primary, secondary and tertiary levels, links with traditional systems of medicine, links with nongovernmental organizations in the health sector, links with national and multilateral donor agencies in the health sector, and links with international agencies such as WHO.

Collaboration outside the health sector involves working with government departments and nongovernmental agencies concerned with housing, employment, social welfare, education and criminal justice among others.

5.6.1 Examples of levels of collaboration

Intersectoral collaboration can take place between the above agencies at various levels.

a) At the most basic level, collaboration can involve mutual data-sharing and information exchange, thus increasing awareness between collaborators.
b) At a higher level, agencies are involved in consultation and planning but specific services are still delivered by a particular agency.
c) More intense collaboration involves agencies working together in the planning and delivery of new services.
d) At the most intense level there are joint funding arrangements and joint managerial responsibilities for specific services that are developed jointly by the collaborating agencies.

Collaboration can take place at various levels.

5.6.2 Enhancing collaboration

The requirements for effective collaboration include, first and foremost, an acceptance by the agencies concerned of the need for collaborative efforts. Mental health agencies and the people involved in the planning and delivery of mental health services have to take a lead in explaining and convincing people in other sectors, especially those outside health, of this need. Some ways of enhancing collaboration include: involving other sectors in policy formulation; delegating responsibility for certain activities to agencies from other sectors; setting up information networks that involve agencies from other sectors; and establishing national advisory committees with representatives of relevant agencies from sectors outside mental health (Box 16).

Agencies can benefit substantially from collaboration.

Box 16. Strategies for enhancing collaboration

The basic areas of collaboration include the exchange of information on: philosophy, policy and the range of ongoing activities; areas of success; existing problems; and areas of need. Personal visits are very effective in building networks and bridges. These should be complemented by meetings, brainstorming workshops, newsletters, telephone conversations, correspondence and the use of web sites where possible.

Policy formulation

Policy formulation should involve as many relevant sectors as possible. Government may decide to delegate the task of collecting ideas and seeking consensus to an agency, e.g. a university institution, with appropriate experience. This might involve, for example, holding a planning meeting with all stakeholders in order to clarify the mental health policy interests of the participants.

Delegation of responsibility

Some government agencies, e.g. regional consultant hospitals, could take up the responsibilities of training and supervising mental health workers in their regions. Professional organizations might take up the function and responsibility of producing educational or training materials for mental health workers. Governments might provide subsidies to voluntary bodies for the purpose of providing mental health services to communities. It is also conventional for governments to establish contracts with institutions or individuals in universities for the monitoring and evaluation of activities in the field of mental health. In many instances this approach is more cost-effective than setting up research organizations in health ministries.

Information and the coordination of mental health programmes

It is important to keep lines of communication open in order to maintain organic coherence between the various sectors involved in mental health promotion. The motivation of all actors and stakeholders requires them to be informed about what is happening all the time. Communication can be maintained through electronic media, briefs and newsletters.

Setting up information and communication strategies or networks

The process of setting up networks, information systems and communication strategies is most likely to follow the policy development process. Stakeholders may have to be involved from the outset, defining what they need to communicate about and how communication can be achieved. The outcome, therefore, is likely to be dictated by the objective situation obtaining in the country concerned.

Establishment of national advisory and coordinating committees

It is important that national planning committees, representing all stakeholders, should define the various advisory committees and their functions as well as their membership. These committees should preferably include representatives of all the stakeholders. Umbrella organizations may represent a number of bodies on these committees in order to keep them small and functional.

Key points: Issues concerning the organization of mental health services

- There is evidence from developed countries that community-based treatments are more effective or at least as effective as hospital-based treatments.

- There is evidence that depression can be successfully treated in primary care settings.

- Mental disorders that run a chronic course or a relapsing remitting course are better managed by services that adopt a continuing care approach, emphasizing the long-term nature of these disorders and the need for ongoing therapeutic input.

- The pathways to care differ in developing and developed countries. Existing pathways may hinder access to care in some instances and may have to be reformed.

- It is necessary to address geographical disparities in the provision of mental health services.

- Mental health services should adopt a needs-led approach.

- The complex needs of persons with mental disorders cut across sectors and cannot be met by the mental health sector alone. Collaboration within the health sector and with other sectors outside the health sector is therefore necessary.

- The first step towards effective collaboration is acknowledgement of the need for it.

- Some ways of enhancing collaboration include: involving other sectors in policy formulation; delegating responsibility for certain activities to agencies from other sectors; setting up information networks involving agencies from other sectors; and establishing national advisory committees representing relevant agencies from sectors outside the mental health sector.

6. Recommendations and conclusions

A number of general recommendations of how services for mental health can be organized to optimise the delivery of high quality care are suggested below. These need to be considered and adapted according to the specific country context.

- If possible, large and centralized psychiatric institutions should be closed down and more appropriate community-based alternatives should be provided. It may not be realistic to take this course immediately in many countries. In the short term these institutions should be reduced in size, the living conditions of the patients should be improved, and staff should be trained to deliver care in the community and improve the quality of care. These institutions should be converted into centres for active treatment and rehabilitation.

- As far as possible, all new admissions to mental hospitals should be stopped. Patients needing admission to hospital should be accommodated in psychiatric units in general hospitals.

- Existing financial and human resources should be diverted from large mental hospitals to mental health care services in primary care and to community-based mental health services.

- The integration of mental health services into primary care and general hospitals should be given priority. Integration forms the basis for reorienting services from the institutional perspective to the community-based perspective.

- In developing countries, specialized mental health services should be made available in general hospital settings at the district level.

- Informal mental health care, provided by families, self-help groups or volunteer workers, should be maximized by improving the general understanding of mental disorders and their causes, the available treatments, and management skills. Support and education groups for families and other carers should be maximized.

- Financial disincentives should be used in order to discourage care in specialized psychiatric institutions, and financial incentives should be used to promote care in general hospitals and the community.

- In developing countries, mental health specialists should be used wisely in the training and supervision of less specialized mental health workers.

- The service provision gap between rural and urban areas, and underprovision in any underserved populations, should be reduced by extending the reach of general health services and community mental health services.

- The training of health care professionals should encompass the psychosocial aspects of care along with skills and knowledge about appropriate medical treatments.

- Consideration should be given to both the short-term and long-term requirements for the training of specialist and general health workers. In developing countries it is justifiable to emphasize the training of general health workers in the short term and in the long term. Attention should also be paid to increasing specialist capacity in the long term.

- The involvement of consumer and family organizations in service planning and delivery should be encouraged and increased.

7. Scenarios for the organization of services in countries with various levels of resources

These scenarios use two fictitious countries similar to those described in *Mental Health Policy, Plans and Programmes*.

Country A with a population of 10 million and a low level of resources

- There are two mental hospitals in the country which limit admission to persons with severe psychosis and disruptive behaviour.
- Outpatient treatment is available only in four cities and covers 40% of the population.
- The country has 20 psychiatrists, 30 psychologists and 80 psychiatric nurses. About 30-50% of their time is spent on private practice and teaching.
- There is a good network of primary care centres and a basic level of primary care is available in nearly all rural and urban areas.

The main aims in organizing services should be to improve access to outpatient and inpatient services throughout the country, especially for people living in rural areas, and to help persons with mental disorders to continue living in the community.

The following steps should be taken.

a) Prioritization should be undertaken in respect of certain mental health conditions. It is important that the community be consulted when priorities are decided so that its perceived needs are addressed. This can be achieved by consulting widely with mental health professionals, community leaders, and people with mental disorders and their families. Two possible outcomes follow from such consultation. The community and the professionals may either identify common mental disorders, i.e. depression and anxiety, that should be prioritized for action because they affect the lives of many people and because the cumulative disability for the population is much greater than that caused by severe mental disorders, or they may decide that severe mental disorders with a chronic course should be prioritized for action because they cause significant disability in the persons concerned, hardship for the families of these persons and disruption to the social life of other community members.

b) The next step should be to ensure that the limited number of mental health professionals is used to obtain maximum benefit. As far as possible, mental health professionals should be used for training, supervision and dealing with referred cases rather than for direct service provision for all persons with mental disorders.

c) Direct services should be provided by primary care workers, who should be trained and supervised by the mental health professionals. The primary care workers should refer specific cases to mental health professionals, who should provide specialist consultations, draw up treatment plans and send patients back to the primary care workers for the implementation of these plans.

d) Admission beds should be made available in as many general hospitals as possible. Each general hospital should therefore have at least one psychiatrist, one psychologist and four psychiatric nurses in its admissions unit. The mental health professionals should also provide a consultation and liaison service to patients admitted for physical disorders.

e) Long-stay patients in the two mental hospitals should be reviewed in order to assess their long-term needs for treatment and care. Assessments should attempt to ascertain the level of support required in order enable the patients to live in the community. As a first step, all new admissions to these two hospitals should be stopped and the patients in question should be directed to the general hospital nearest to their home for admission.

A clear plan should be drawn up for discharging patients from these hospitals over a period of five years. This process should start with those patients with the least disability and with families who are willing to take them home. Ongoing treatment of the patients' mental disorders should be handed over to local primary care centres and provision should be made for periodic reviews of their treatment by mental health professionals at the general hospitals nearest to their places of residence.
f) Training should be started for staff working in other health programmes, e.g. in the HIV/AIDS programme, and for health care staff involved in providing reproductive and child health services.

Country B with a population of 10 million and a medium level of resources

- Some primary care centres deliver basic treatment for mental disorders and one nongovernmental organization has a programme on life skills and the school health environment.
- Most mental health resources are concentrated in two cities: there are two inpatient units in general hospitals and there is a large mental hospital.
- There are 100 psychiatrists, 40 psychologists, 250 psychiatric nurses and 40 occupational therapists.

The main aim in the organization of services is to extend access to them to underserved populations, especially in rural areas.

This country should take the following steps.

a) The mental health conditions that are to be addressed should be prioritized (see country A above).
b) All primary care centres, especially those in rural areas, should deliver basic treatment for mental disorders. This requires all the staff in primary care centres to receive training in mental health and continuing weekly supervision by mental health professionals.
c) Some mental health professionals should devote a significant part of their working time to dealing with specialist referrals from primary care staff.
d) Outpatient clinics should be started in all primary care centres. These clinics should initially function as specialist clinics and should be held once a week. Psychotropic medications should be made available in all primary centres.
e) Referral links should be set up between primary care centres and psychiatric units in general hospitals. This process may be aided by dividing the country into sectors and identifying the catchment area for each psychiatric unit. Primary care centres in the catchment area of a general hospital's psychiatric unit, should refer patients to, and receive supervision from, the mental health professionals in that unit.
f) Inpatient psychiatric beds should be set up in all general hospitals. General hospitals in rural areas or other areas where access is poor should be prioritized for funding and human resources.
g) There should be collaboration with the nongovernmental organization in order to provide services for children and adolescents. Members of staff of the nongovernmental organization should be trained to identify mental disorders and to acquire basic counselling skills.
h) A plan should be implemented for gradually reducing the number of beds in the large psychiatric hospital (see country A above).

8. Barriers and solutions

Some of the barriers hindering the organization of mental health services are discussed below and ways of overcoming them are suggested. The solutions indicated are not necessarily the only ones that might be applied in order to achieve effective and appropriate mental health services.

Barrier 1

Primary care staff receiving skills training in the field of mental health may not necessarily apply their newly acquired knowledge in the course of their duties. In Guinea-Bissau, for example, primary care workers did not apply their skills to the identification and treatment of major mental disorders on their own initiative (De Jong, 1996).

Problems of motivating primary care staff to apply their training in the field of mental health.

Solutions

1. Regular supervision and consultation with a designated team of mental health professionals was effective for primary care nurses in Guinea-Bissau.

Regular supervision.

2. Resistance to providing psychosocial counselling may be attributable to a cultural reluctance to discuss emotional issues frankly, a continued belief in the somatic basis of many minor mental ailments, or the attribution of the symptoms to a traditional supernatural factor on the part of both primary care workers and patients. The primary care nurses in this example may have required additional training to address the need for psychosocial counselling. The example of Zimbabwe (Abas et al., 1995; Patel, 2000) suggests that community-oriented research using key informants could help to identify common local idiomatic forms of minor mental ailments and generate recommendations for treatment. These should form the basis of a culturally relevant diagnosis and treatment programme offered by primary care nurses. The educational component should consist of learning to identify and treat these idiomatic forms of minor mental disorders on the basis of using the information gathered from both nurses and the community.

Use local idiomatic forms of mental illness as the basis of training.

3. Cambodia represents the inverse of the problem found in Guinea-Bissau, viz. the resistance of some local mental health trainers to incorporating traditional concepts into the mental health training package (Somasundaram et al., 1999). The solution is similar to that in the example from Guinea-Bissau in that it requires demonstrating to local health workers how local idiomatic forms of mental illness complement or coincide with Western categories of mental disorder. Cross-cultural issues should therefore form an explicit component of the skills training package.

Demonstrate the correspondence between local and Western categories of mental illness.

Barrier 2

Geographically large countries that are poor and have predominantly rural populations may find it difficult to establish workable networks of mental health services at the level of primary care because of a lack of financial and human resources in outlying primary care clinics.

Geographically large countries may have difficulty in implementing coordinated mental health services at the primary care level.

Solutions

The example of Botswana illustrates that psychiatric nurses who regularly visit remote rural primary care clinics represent a cost-effective way of spreading scarce mental health personnel over vast geographical regions (Ben-Tovim, 1987). The use of psychiatric nurses would be even more effective if village-level mental health workers aided them in identifying vulnerable cases in the community. Such mental health workers should identify patients and refer them to local primary care clinics on the days when psychiatric nurses make their visits. Another possibility would be to train volunteer village community mental health workers on the basis of the core-group trainer concept (Somasundaram et al., 1999).

Regular visits of psychiatric nurses to designated primary care clinics.

Training for village-level community health workers.

Barrier 3

For many countries the provision of adequate cost-effective mental health services can be maximized through an increasing emphasis on intersectoral cooperation. However, this is by no means a straightforward process.

A lack of intersectoral cooperation impedes the development of innovative and cost-effective mental health services.

Solutions

1. The examples of Tanzania (Kilonzo & Simmons, 1998), Zimbabwe (Abas et al., 1995), Cambodia (Somasundaram et al., 1999) and India (Box 6) illustrate that cooperative approaches can occur at the national or local level and can bring together local community members, service providers and social agencies. Cooperation between mental health services, general health services, traditional healers and community members is very important, leading to the development of cost-effective and appropriate primary-level mental health services.

Programmes that forge links between mental health services, general health services, traditional healers and local communities.

2. Services such as psychiatric agricultural rehabilitation villages and counselling for depression in primary care are structured on the basis of a network of cooperation between mental health services and various other sectors. These services are products of intersectoral cooperation, and in developing countries it may be helpful to think of the mental health system as a collaborator with other sectors in providing personnel

Coordinate a collaboration network in order to provide mental health services.

(psychiatrists, psychiatric nurses, primary care nurses, medical attendants, traditional healers, teachers, village health workers, etc.), services (psychiatry, primary care, traditional healing, education), and service items (pharmacotherapy, counselling, herbal cures, relaxation and meditation exercises).

Barrier 4

Failure of services to detect people with mental disorders because of fragmented care, ignorance and poor communication on mental health.

Existing services often obstruct the early detection and treatment of mental disorders. The late entry of users into the specialist mental health system is often attributable to previous ineffective contacts with traditional or primary care providers. This occurs for the following reasons.

1. There may be a lack of knowledge among rural populations concerning the causes of and treatments for mental disorders.

2. A lack of mental health training and of coordination of activities between traditional healers, primary care staff and mental health professionals may contribute to the absence of early detection and treatment at the primary care level.

3. Primary care personnel may remain in clinics or offices instead of actively visiting communities in order to promote mental health and identify persons with mental disorders who are in need of treatment.

Solutions

Active health education and early identification in communities at the primary care level lead to improved outcomes and a reduction in the cost of care.

1. Apart from specialized training for primary care staff, countries with a more active community approach to care, e.g. the Czech Republic and India, have established better communication with local communities and have thus made the pathways to mental health services more readily visible. Where community health workers and primary care workers actively promote health education and early identification in communities, vulnerable persons and their families are more likely than would otherwise be the case to know about and use mental health services as opposed to traditional healers.

2. Lines of communication can be improved if:

(a) home visits are made by community health workers and general practitioners;
(b) regular meetings are held with community members such as teachers, religious leaders and traditional healers;
(c) there is community screening for major mental disorders on the basis of an assessment scale

such as that of the general health questionnaire (Breakey, 1996c).

3. A reciprocal network of communication for primary care staff and specialist mental health services at the secondary and tertiary levels is required for complex cases of severe mental disorders or comorbid disorders.

A reciprocal consultation network involving all three levels of service provision.

Barrier 5

In many countries, mental health funding, personnel and services are concentrated in tertiary-level institutions. In contrast, a community-oriented approach emphasizes:

(1) dedicated services for population groups;
(2) multidisciplinary personnel;
(3) treatment close to people's homes, with minimal disruption of family and social networks,
in preference to chronic institutional settings.

The concentration of financial and human resources in tertiary mental health institutions.

However, medically trained mental health staff and the administrative bureaucracies responsible for the organization of mental health services often resist this decentralized community approach to service provision (Gallegos & Montero, 1999; Rezaki et al., 1995; Tomov, 1999).

Resistance to changing to community care among mental health and administrative staff.

Solutions

1. Staff resistance to a shift in resources to secondary-level and primary-level settings in the community can be overcome by restructuring the teaching curriculum so that it includes community and public health approaches to the management of mental health issues.

Restructure the teaching curriculum so that it embraces a public health approach to mental health.

2. A concerted effort at national level to involve existing tertiary-level staff in structural change is required. If the roles of personnel are not diminished but redefined with their cooperation, resistance to a shift in resource allocation is likely to be less than would otherwise be the case. For example, psychiatrists, psychologists and psychiatric nurses can take on a variety of roles ranging from direct clinical care to planning and consultation.

The roles of tertiary-level staff can be redefined in relation to clinical, planning and consultative functions.

3. The example of the former Eastern Bloc countries indicates that both mental health staff and centralized administrations often resist a shift in service priorities even though gaps in service provision are recognized by users and newly elected governments (Tomov, 1999). In this context, governments may wish to side-step centralized bureaucracies by switching funds to nongovernmental organizations or other non-profit

Shift funds from tertiary providers to nongovernmental organizations, primary care or community-orientated mental health services.

service providers that offer decentralized community-oriented mental health services at the secondary and primary care levels. In the Czech Republic, for example, FOKUS, a nongovernmental organization providing various mental health services, receives funding from several government ministries (Holmes & Koznar, 1998).

4. Intersectoral collaboration between government ministries, private non-profit service providers and nongovernmental organization providers can be expected to become increasingly important in shifting resources from tertiary to secondary and primary mental health services in communities.

Intersectoral cooperation is vital in order to shift resources from the tertiary level to other levels of mental health care.

Barrier 6

Some developing countries possess more community residential and outpatient mental health services than others. Nevertheless, few developing countries have a sufficiency of these services in their rural regions, and community services may be inadequate for children, adolescents and the elderly in urban or rural regions.

Barrier 6

Scarce community mental health services.

Solutions

1. Human and financial resources should be shifted from institutional settings at the tertiary and secondary levels to community settings at the secondary and primary levels of service provision. The examples of countries that have managed this change (e.g. India, Israel) indicate that it can occur through national or regional initiatives involving:

- resource allocation;
- staff training;
- follow-up of trained staff;
- intersectoral cooperation with families of users, community members, other categories of health workers, and education and social services.

Solutions

National and regional planning initiatives for resource allocation, staff training, performance evaluation and intersectoral cooperation.

The development of community mental health services requires the cooperation of service providers and health department personnel.

2. Without strong government interest in the provision of community alternatives to institutional mental health services, little progress can be made beyond a private niche market in urban settings. This is particularly true in relation to mental health services for children, adolescents and elderly people who require special provision in the areas of policy legislation, staff training and budget allocations.

Community mental health services for children, adolescents and elderly people require government commitment and special provision at the national or regional level.

Barrier 7

Some countries have attempted to shift the provision of mental health services to the primary level of care, i.e. with programmes aimed at integrating mental health services into a pre-existing primary care network catering for physical health. These attempts have encountered many barriers.

- General practitioners, nurses and community health workers located in primary care centres usually lack training in mental health despite being the first line of consultation for patients with mental problems. The same is true of general practitioners in private practice.
- Without sustained skills training and active follow-up of primary care staff, the integration of a mental health component into the detection and management of mental health problems is unlikely to occur.
- Consultations last only about five minutes in many developing and developed countries. Consequently, much of the mental health skills training received by primary care workers is wasted, as little in the way of knowledge or services can be operationalized in such a short time.
- General practitioners do not always have long-term continuity with individual patients and may not communicate with family members or traditional healers about mental health problems in the community.

Barrier 7

Problems in providing mental health services in primary care settings.

Solutions

1. The solution to the first two points lies in changing the emphasis of training for primary care workers and in constructing a sound consultation and referral network that enables easy access to mental health professionals at the secondary and tertiary levels of care. The training of established primary care teams should preferably occur in the settings where they see patients, and should involve simple steps in the diagnosis and management of both common and severe mental disorders.

2. The training of new primary care staff in the field of mental health requires a change in emphasis from an institutional psychiatry model to a community-based public health model (Ozturk, 2000).

3. One possible solution is to link mental health needs with general health concerns that have a higher national priority but are nevertheless very relevant to mental health, e.g. AIDS. This enables funding to become available for the training of primary care staff in a variety of mental health skills. For example, the need for counselling skills within the framework of an AIDS prevention programme has resulted in the

Solutions

The training of established primary care teams should occur in service settings and should involve programmes in diagnosis, management, and follow-up consultations.

The mental health sector should link its own initiatives with general health priorities in order to obtain funding for primary mental health care services.

appropriate skills training of primary care personnel in South Africa (Freeman, 2000). In the context of primary care the mental health sector should work in close cooperation with the general health sector at the national level in order to take advantage of such training opportunities. Other linkages between specialist mental health and general health concerns could include the integration of:

- a children's mental health component into mother and child health care;
- an adolescent mental health component into AIDS and substance abuse programmes;
- child and adolescent mental health concerns into health education in schools;
- a geriatric mental health component into programmes for family health and home visits.

4. The problems of brief consultation periods in primary care in some countries could be solved by a more active approach to early identification in the community. This would save the time of general practitioners in making diagnoses and would enable them to set up management programmes whereby follow-up would be performed by health workers. In India, where primary care workers already visit local communities in connection with general health issues (Channabasavanna et al., 1995), mental health promotion and early identification could be integrated into these activities. This would make the diagnostic and management tasks of general practitioners more feasible in the limited time available for consultation.

Active mental health promotion and early identification by primary or local community mental health workers.

5. If the national model of primary care involves impersonal clinical care by general practitioners and no continuity of personal contacts between patients and doctors (Üstün & Von Korff, 1995), community health workers or nurses from clinics should conduct periodic follow-up visits with patients in their community settings.

Barrier 8

Many countries have fewer mental health resources in rural settings than in urban settings. This is especially the case for all tertiary services and specialist child, adolescent and geriatric services. In addition, the need to shift financial and human resources from tertiary to secondary and primary care in community settings (see barrier 5 above) there is also a need to shift such resources from urban settings to rural areas. The solution to the first issue may result in urban areas developing an array of secondary and primary community mental health services while remote rural regions remain without comparable resources and

Barrier 8

The urban bias: there are fewer human and infrastructural resources for mental health services in rural areas.

services. Shifting funds to rural areas may not result in significant numbers of mental health professionals moving to these regions, which is a major problem for mental health services that rely heavily on human resources. A significant shift of mental health infrastructure from urban to rural areas is unlikely to occur in most developing countries because of the financial constraints on national health budgets.

Solutions

1. The training of local community workers who can assume some of the responsibility for the early identification of vulnerable community members and participate in the long-term management of such patients after consultation with primary care general practitioners or nurses. Skill components may include attention to the developmentally different mental health needs of children, adolescents and the elderly.

Train rural community health workers in early identification and attention to the developmental needs of children, adolescents and the elderly.

2. Mental health skills training for rural schoolteachers in order to provide health promotion and early identification of mental health issues for children and adolescents.

Train rural schoolteachers in mental health promotion and the early identification of children and adolescents.

3. Mental health skills training for local village and religious leaders including components relating to children, adolescents and the elderly.

Train rural village and religious leaders in health promotion and care of the elderly.

4. Mental health skills training for primary health care workers and their ongoing consultation and follow-up by mental health specialists were discussed above (see Barrier 7).

Barrier 9

National insensitivity to the need for intersectoral approaches

Despite the relative scarcity of mental health services in many countries, particularly in rural regions, there have been few sustained attempts to integrate a mental health component into primary care. Furthermore, community residential and outpatient services are poor in rural areas in both developed and developing countries. A major obstacle to planning for primary mental health care and community services is a lack of initiative at the national level for achieving cooperation between mental health care, primary care, and other sectors involved in mental health, e.g. those of education, social services, correctional services, nongovernmental organizations and donor agencies.

- If cooperation between these sectors is absent at the national level it is comparatively difficult for it to occur at the tertiary, secondary and primary levels of service provision.

- The effectiveness and accessibility of available mental health services may be compromised by a lack of intersectoral cooperation at the point of service provision.

- Different government ministries may run similar psychosocial programmes without coordinating or streamlining their resources.

- There may be a lack of coordination between service providers and social agencies working with target populations, e.g. the police, correctional services, social welfare, education and organized religion.

- A lack of coordination between mental health services and important informal sector participants may occur, e.g. families of people with mental disorders and traditional healers. This deficiency reduces the visibility and accessibility of services to the target group of potential users.

Solutions

1. The examples of India (Box 6) and Israel (Box 9) suggest that regional or national governments should initiate intersectoral approaches to filling gaps in mental health services at all levels of care.

2. Intersectoral approaches should begin with cooperation at the national or regional level between government departments and the providers of mental health services, including public, nongovernmental organization and private for-profit providers.

3. An intersectoral approach can be replicated at the different levels of care by emphasizing the importance of the consultation network.

4. At the tertiary level this network includes mental health specialists forging links with related specialist fields in their own institutions. It also includes the forging of links with regional representatives of the police, education and social welfare sectors, non-governmental organizations and insurers in connection with the planning and implementation of specialist services, e.g. for children, adolescents and elderly people.

5. At the secondary level the network includes mental health workers consulting other sectors, including local municipal representatives of the police, education, organized religion, other social services and non-governmental organizations. The consultations should cover the coordination, planning and implementation of community mental health facilities and rehabilitation services. In addition it is desirable to consult regularly

Solutions

Regional or national governments should initiate intersectoral action to fill gaps in mental health services.

Cooperation between government departments and all mental health service providers.

Cooperation between tertiary providers, regional government departments, nongovernmental organizations and insurers in planning specialist services.

Cooperation between secondary providers, local government departments, nongovernmental organizations and community and religious leaders in planning community mental health services.

with the families of people who have mental disorders and with traditional healers.

6. At the primary level the network includes consultations with local community health workers and individual contacts with local police, teachers, clerics, nongovernmental organizations, family members and traditional healers. These consultations should cover the coordination, planning and implementation of primary mental health education, the prevention of mental disorders and the promotion of programmes in community settings.

Cooperation between primary providers, local institutions, nongovernmental organizations and individuals from communities in the implementation of programmes for the promotion of mental health and the prevention of mental disorders.

9. Glossary

Closed institutions / Institutions whose working is not open to scrutiny and inspection by outside agencies, and which do not encourage such scrutiny. The term does not refer to institutions that have closed down and are non-functional.

Double funding or hump funding / The provision of financial resources for operating an existing service and a new service during a transitional period when there may be an overlap in respect of the services provided and the group or groups served. The ultimate aim is to terminate the existing service once the new service is fully operational and able to meet the needs of the identified target group or groups.

Indirect costs / Costs, apart from direct service costs, incurred by people with mental disorders and their families. For example, people with mental disorders may have to pay for transport so that they can travel long distances to services, or they may lose income as a result of having to spend time away from work while they attend clinics. Families may lose income if family members have to stay at home and care for persons with mental disorders.

Revolving door syndrome / A cycle of admission to hospital, discharge and readmission. This may happen, for instance, because of non-adherence to medications or a lack of follow-up by community-based services, with the result that patients with mental disorders experience relapses.

Stand-alone services / Mental health services that generally function in isolation and do not have strong links with the rest of the health care system. They have little interdependence or reliance on other parts of the health system for meeting the needs of their patients.

References

1. Abas M et al. (1995) Health service and community-based responses to mental ill-health in urban areas. In: Harpham T, Blue I, eds. *Urbanization and mental health in developing countries*, Avebury, Aldershot.

2. Ahmed AM et al. (1996) Capabilities of public, voluntary and private dispensaries in basic health service provision. *World Health Forum*, 17:257-60.

3. Alem A et al. (1999) How are mental disorders seen and where is help sought in a rural Ethiopian community? *Acta Psychiatrica Scandinavica*, 100:40-7.

4. Alves DN, Valentini W (2002) Mental health policy in Brazil. In: Morrall PA, Hazelton M, eds. *Mental health policy: international perspectives*. London: Whurr.

5. Awas M, Kedebe D, Alem A (1999) Major mental disorders in Butajira, southern Ethiopia. *Acta Psychiatrica Scandinavica*, 100:56-64.

6. Barrientos G (2001) La Reorientación de la Atención Psiquiátrica en Cuba. In: *Enfoques para un debate en salud mental colectivo de autores*. Havana: Ediciones Conexiones. p. 87-137. (In Spanish.)

7. Ben-Tovim DJ (1987) *Development psychiatry: mental health and primary health care in Botswana*. London: Tavistock Publications.

8. Bertolote JM (1992) Planificación y administración de acciones en salud mental en la comunidad. In: Levav I, ed. *Temas de salud mental en la comunidad*. Washington DC: OPS. (PALTEX Series No. 19.) (In Spanish.)

9. Bower P et al. (2000) Randomised controlled trial of non-directive counselling cognitive behaviour therapy, and usual general practitioner care for patients with depression. II: Cost-effectiveness. *British Medical Journal*, 321:1389-92.

10. Braun P et al. (1981) Overview of psychiatric patients: a critical review of outcome studies. *American Journal of Psychiatry*, 136:736.

11. Breakey WR (1996a) Inpatient services. In: Breakey WR, ed. *Integrated mental health services*. New York: Oxford University Press Inc. p. 264-75.

12. Breakey WR (1996b) The catchment area. In: Breakey WR, ed. *Integrated mental health services*. New York: Oxford University Press Inc. p. 139-45.

13. Breakey WR (1996c) Developmental milestones for community psychiatry. In: Breakey WR, ed. *Integrated mental health services*. New York: Oxford University Press Inc. p. 29-42.

14. Channabasavanna SM, Sriram TG, Kumar K (1995) Results from the Bangalore center. In: Üstün TB, Sartorius N, eds. *Mental illness in general health care: an international study*. Chichester JohnWiley and Sons. p. 79-97.

15. Collins PY et al. (1999a) Using local resources in Patagonia: primary care and mental health in Neuquen, Argentina. *International Journal of Mental Health*, 28:3-16.

16. Collins PY et al. (1999b) Using local resources in Patagonia: a model of community-based rehabilitation. *International Journal of Mental Health*, 28:17-24.

17. Conway M et al. (1994) *A companion to purchasing mental health services*. Cambridge: Anglia and Oxford Regional Health Authority.

18. Cooper PJ, Murray L (1998) Postnatal depression. *British Medical Journal*, 316:1884-6.

19. De Jong JTVM (1996) A comprehensive public mental health programme in Guinea-Bissau: a useful model for African, Asian and Latin-American countries. *Psychological Medicine*, 26:97-108.

20. Dixon LB, Lehman AF (1995) Family interventions for schizophrenia. *Schizophrenia Bulletin*, 21(4):631-43.

21. Freeman M (2000) Using all opportunities for improving mental health examples from South Africa. *Bulletin of the World Health Organization*, 78:508-10.

22. Gallegos A, Montero F (1999) Issues in community-based rehabilitation for persons with mental illness in Costa Rica. *International Journal of Mental Health*, 28:25-30.

23. Goldberg DP, Lecrubier Y (1995) Form and frequency of mental disorders across centres. In: Üstün TB, Sartorius N, eds. *Mental illness in general health care: an international study*. Chichester: John Wiley and Sons 323B334.

24. Goodwin S (1997) *Comparative mental health policy: from institutional to community care*. London: Sage Publications.

25. Gureje O et al. (1995) Results from the Ibadan center. In: Üstün TB, Sartorius N, eds. *Mental illness in general health care: an international study*. Chichester: John Wiley and Sons. p. 157-73.

26. Holmes T, Koznar J (1998) The impact of independence on the development of community mental health services in the Czech Republic. *International Journal of Mental Health*, 27:18-45.

27. Jacob KS (2001) Community care for people with mental disorders in developing countries. Problems and possible solutions. *British Journal of Psychiatry*, 178:296-8.

28. Ji J (1995) Advances in mental health services in Shanghai, China. *International Journal of Mental Health*, 23:90-7.

29. Kilonzo GP, Simmons N (1998) Development of mental health services in Tanzania: a reappraisal for the future. *Social Science and Medicine*, 47:419-28.

30. Leff J, Gamble C (1995) Training of community psychiatric nurses in family work for schizophrenia. *International Journal of Mental Health*, 24:76–88.

31. Levkoff SE, Macarthur IW, Bucknall J (1995) Elderly mental health in the developing world. *Social Science and Medicine*, 41:983-1003.

32. Mohit A et al. (1999) Mental health manpower development in Afghanistan: Report of a training course for primary health care physicians. *Eastern Mediterranean Health Journal*, 5(2):215-9.

33. Mubbashar MH (1999) Mental health services in rural Pakistan. In: Tansella M. Thornicroft G, eds. *Common mental disorders in primary care - Essays in honour of Professor Sir David Goldberg*. London: Routledge.

34. Murthy SR (1998) Rural psychiatry in developing countries. *Psychiatric Services*, 49:967-9.

35. Murthy SR (2000) Community resources for mental health care in India. *Epidemiologia e Psychiatria Sociale*, 9(2):89-92.

36. Mynors-Wallis L (1996) Problem solving treatment: evidence for effectiveness and feasibility in primary care. *International Journal of Psychiatric Medicine*, 26:249-62.

37. Nikapota AD (1991) Child psychiatry in developing countries. *British Journal of Psychiatry*, 158:743-51.

38. Ozturk MO (2000) Removing the barriers to effective mental health care: a view from Turkey. *Bulletin of the World Health Organization*, 78:506-7.

39. Patel V (2000) Health systems research: a pragmatic model for meeting mental health needs in low-income countries. In: Andrews G, Henderson S, eds. *Unmet need in psychiatry: problems, resources, responses*. Cambridge: Cambridge University Press. p. 363-77.

40. Pearson V (1992) Community and culture: a Chinese model of community care for the mentally ill. *International Journal of Social Psychiatry*, 38:163-78.

41. Rezaki MS et al. (1995) Results from the Ankara center. In: Üstün TB, Sartorius N, eds. *Mental illness in general health care: an international study*. Chichester: John Wiley and Sons. p. 39-55.

42. Schulberg HC et al. (1996) Treating major depression in primary care practice: eight-month clinical outcomes. *Archives of General Psychiatry*, 53:913–9.

43. Sidandi P et al. (1999) Psychiatric rehabilitation: the perspective from Botswana. *International Journal of Mental Health*, 28:31-7.

44. Somasundaram DJ et al. (1999) Starting mental health services in Cambodia. *Social Science and Medicine*, 48:1029-46.

45. Sriram TG et al. (1990) Training primary care medical officers in mental health care: an evaluation using a multiple choice questionnaire. *Acta Psychiatrica Scandinavica*, 81: 414-7.

46. Talbott JA (1978) *The death of the asylum: a critical study of state hospital management, services, and care*. New York: Grune and Stratton.

47. Tausig M, Subedi S (1997) The modern mental health system in Nepal: organizational persistence in the absence of legitimating myths. *Social Science and Medicine*, 45:441-7.

48. Thornicroft G, Tansella M (1999) *The mental health matrix: a manual to improve services*. Cambridge: Cambridge University Press.

49. Tomov T (1999) Central and Eastern European countries. In: Thornicroft G, Tansella M, eds. *The mental health matrix: a manual to improve services*. Cambridge: Cambridge University Press. p. 216-27.

50. Trisnantoro L (2002) *Decentralization policy on public mental hospitals in Indonesia: a financial perspective*. Paper presented at the seminar on Mental Health and Health Policy in Developing Countries (15 May 2002). Harvard University.

51. Tyano S, Mozes T (1998) Mental health reform: the Israeli experience. In: Young JG, Ferrari P, eds. *Designing mental health services and systems for children and adolescents: A shrewd investment*. Philadelphia: Brunner/Mazel. p. 295-304.

52. Üstün TB, Sartorius N (1995) *Mental illness in general health care: an international study*. Chichester: John Wiley and Sons.

53. Üstün TB, Von Korff M (1995) Primary mental health services: access and provision of care. In Üstün TB, Sartorius N, eds. *Mental illness in general health care: an international study*. Chichester: John Wiley and Sons. p. 347-60.

54. Ward E et al. (2000) Randomised controlled trial of non-directive counselling, cognitive behaviour therapy and usual general practitioner care for patients with depression. I: clinical effectiveness. *British Medical Journal*, 321:1381-8.

55. World Health Organization (1982) *Training in mental health for primary health care workers*. Report of a workshop for trainers in mental health for nurses, medical assistants and village health workers. Maseru, 30 March to 10 April 1981 (unpublished document AFR/MH/12. This document is available from the WHO Regional Office for Africa).

56. World Health Organization (2000) *Making a difference in Mongolian mental health: the Nations for Mental Health Project of the WHO to reorient mental health in Mongolia*, 1997-2000. Geneva: World Health Organization.

57. World Health Organization (2001a) *World health report 2001. Mental health: new understanding, new hope*. Geneva: World Health Organization.

58. World Health Organization (2001b) *Atlas: Mental health resources in the world*. Geneva: World Health Organization.

59. World Health Organization (2001) *Innovative care for chronic conditions: building blocks for action: global report*. Geneva: World Health Organization (unpublished document WHO/NMH/CCH/01. This report is available from the Department "Management of Noncommunicable Diseases" at WHO CH-1211, Geneva 27, Switzerland. It can also be accessed through the internet at "The Observatory on Health Care for Chronic Conditions" at the following link: http://www.who.int/chronic_conditions/en/)

60. Yan HQ, Xiao SF, Lu YF (1995) Results from the Shanghai center. In Üstün TB, Sartorius N, eds. *Mental illness in general health care: an international study*. Chichester: John Wiley and Sons. p. 285-300.

61. Yousaf F (1997) Psychiatry in Pakistan. *International Journal of Social Psychiatry*, 43:298-302.